Medicine
of the
Future

The Patient-Centered Approach
to Coordinating Effective Medical Care

Dr. Brandie Gowey, NMD

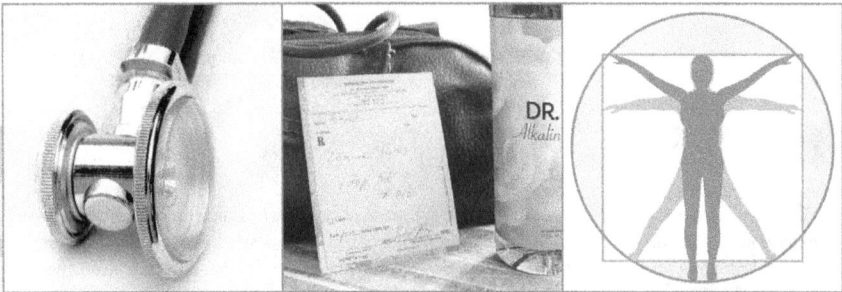

with foreword by
Dr. James Carter, MD

❧ Edited by ❧
Dr. Daphne Cornman, NMD

Charlotte Fox   Jan Zoucha   Dianna Hales

Medicine of the Future
The Patient-Centered Approach
to Coordinating Effective Medical Care

Published by
DR. DNA Press
Flagstaff, AZ

Printed in the United States of America

ISBN: 978-0-9861850-0-7

Cover and Book Design by
Andi Kleinman

*Proceeds from the sale of this book benefit
medical research at DR. DNA Clinic.
Learn more at **goweyresearchgroup.com**.*

*This book is dedicated
to my grandfather.*

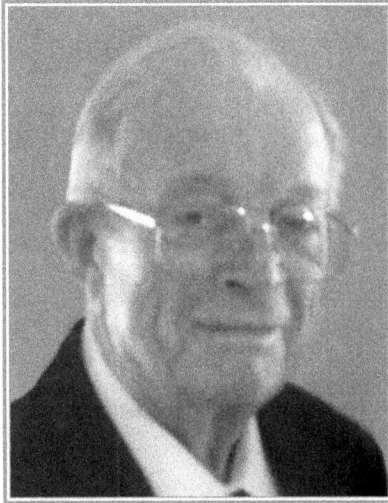

Robert Keyes

❧ Table of Contents ❧

❧ Preface ❧

This book is meant to be a reference guide for you and your family. In my experience, patients feel very overwhelmed or distraught when they go to their physician for their medical concerns. The feelings come from fear at not knowing all the treatment options, or what it really means to seek care that compliments Conventionally offered medicine. Conversely, I have seen Alternative Medicine Practitioners not explain well enough the options or reasons herbs are used over medications.

Many times, because of the lack of education on behalf of the patient, choices are made that lead to very expensive doctor or supplement bills. I am hoping this book can be used to prevent this. Reach for this manual when you are not sure what to expect in terms of options for your diagnosis.

❦ Foreword ❧

Dr. James Carter, MD, Interventional Cardiologist

In her latest book, Dr. Gowey educates the reader about biological systems and their relationship to health and wellness. She explores traditional concepts of healthcare delivery, examining the styles and focus of Conventional Medicine, Alternative Medicine and Naturopathic Medicine. This allows the reader to make better choices as to how to capture the healing power of the body.

I am both a Board-Certified Internist and General/Interventional Cardiologist trained in "traditional" approaches to healthcare delivery at State University of New York Downstate Medical Center, University of Chicago Hospitals, and University of Maryland Medical Center. Even though I am a specialist trained in Conventional Medicine, I have always felt that more collaboration is needed—across disciplines—to help patients the most.

Specialization has led to compartmentalization that does not match the nature of our body's biological systems. Everything in the body is interconnected. Not only do we need specialists who have an enhanced knowledge of particular organ systems and thus disease processes, but also providers who are skilled at addressing the body holistically. Naturopathic Medicine fills this role. Dr. Gowey explains what Naturopathic Medicine brings to the table, how Naturopaths focus on identifying causes of disease and illness, with their mission to empower patients to take control of their health and their bodies. In my field of cardiology, we cannot treat the heart without considering the brain, the liver, the adrenal glands, the kidneys...and vice versa. Specialized care has become compartmentalized care, which is often incomplete care. Is this an out-of-control train that has left the station with no turning back? I think not. Dr. Gowey thinks not.

In *Medicine of the Future*, Dr. Gowey takes on the prevalent misunderstanding of what Naturopathic Medicine is, differentiating it from both Conventional and Alternative Medicine. She explains the differences between these approaches to medical care, using case vignettes and excerpts from communications from patients to highlight her methods and successes.

Although Conventional Medical training does put an emphasis on prevention, it is often not a core value for most practitioners, and not actualized by others. The pressures of volume-based compensation, legal-defensive medicine, and time consuming, inefficient record keeping, are some of the causes of this disconnect. Too many practitioners focus on the use of toxic drugs (pay attention to their disclaimers and warnings!) to treat symptoms and too little time on identifying and treating the cause of the patient's problem. Dr. Gowey deftly explains the fallacy of that approach. The nature of my practice is that patients often come to me severely ill—I must aggressively address the symptoms. It is comforting to work in concert with a Naturopathic Doctor focused on the cause of illness. Once the cause is identified, recurrences can often be prevented.

Dr. Gowey has a vision to incorporate the principles of Naturopathic Medicine (identify and remove obstacles to self-healing, focus on the cause of illness, treat the whole person) with the discipline of Conventional Medicine (pursuing diagnoses, symptom relief, focusing on disease management), both dedicated to doing no harm. This alignment will allow these physicians to work collaboratively, seamlessly, and efficiently to help all of us tap into the immense capacity of the human body to secure optimum health. We need to eliminate the boundaries separating these important fields of medicine. Side-by-side. Collaborative. Efficient. Successful. Find the cause and relate it to the patient. Dr. Gowey has given us a blueprint to build this new healthcare paradigm. The medicine of the future will be all about the patient, not the disease.

❧ Introduction ❧

True "cure" or resolution of symptoms begins with treating the person, not the disease (Banerjee 1931).

Recently, I received a call from a concerned parent regarding her daughter who was suffering from a rash on her face. The mother wanted herbs or a homeopathic remedy as treatment for her daughter and wondered if I could find the right natural medicine.

I explained that I never prescribed medicines until I had a better idea of what may be causing the symptoms; not knowing the root cause(s) inhibits my ability to prescribe or recommend the right medicine(s).

Naturopathic Medicine works on a level focusing on the treatment of causes of diseases and symptoms. Naturopathy follows these principles (Gowey 2014):

First, Do No Harm

Find and utilize treatments that are safe, noninvasive, and have minimal risks.

The Healing Power of Nature

Your body has the ability to heal if given the right nutrients and support.

Find the Cause

Focus on identification and treatment of causes
(the "Obstacle to Cure", Hahnemann 1921) of the disease or condition.

Treat the Whole Person

Everyone has unique genetics, biochemistry, lifestyles, and life experiences. Understanding this in each person allows the physician to develop individualized treatment plans.

Prevention

Prevent health problems and diseases before they start.

The word doctor is Latin for "*to teach*". Your Naturopathic Physician is here to educate you about your body, your health, and your choices.

The medicine of the future will be that which focuses on identifying and treating causes of disease and utilizing the power of the body to bring about healing. This medicine exists in the NOW. It is called Naturopathy and I believe that someday every physician will practice according to these principles.

It has been through the application of these principles that I have learned two additional ideas as they relate to the practice of medicine:

PATIENTS HAVE TO BELIEVE THEIR BODY CAN HEAL

and then...

THEY HAVE TO PUT ACTION BEHIND THEIR BELIEF.

When I sit down with a patient, I open my energy to be able to sense what they need in the NOW. I have noticed that those who set aside fear and are willing to invest in themselves are those who improve the most: these patients want to get better, trust the healing process, and trust their body will know what to do. They are motivated to make the changes they need in order to get better and they **BELIEVE** they will see improvement.

There is a patient who first came to me in May of 2013 who had sustained a work-related spinal injury that forced her to go on disability. The injury caused degeneration of her thoracic spine that was very painful for her.

Even though she was in so much pain and her situation looked hopeless, she decided to **BELIEVE** for healing, and I am happy to report that with prolotherapy (from Dr. Tallman, DC, NMD, www.arizonaprolotherapy.com), acupuncture, vitamin IV therapies, and an anti-inflammatory diet, by month six she was much improved.

She pursued her care, maintained a grateful attitude, treated the causes of her symptoms, supported her body's ability to heal, and she **BELIEVED**. She showed up. She showed up to her appointments even if she was weeping with pain. She showed up and Dr. Tallman and I did too; between the three of us she began to flourish rather than flounder.

If you believe and if you trust your healthcare provider, the energy will show up for everything you need. Even if you struggle with something serious, if you **BELIEVE**, then something will still improve. If you need money to pay for your care, it will show up. If you need to find the right doctor for your care, the right one will show up. If you need a ride to your appointments, someone will offer.

You don't have to be attached to any outcome or anyone or anything about your health:

YOU JUST HAVE TO HOLD
THE ATTITUDE AND ENERGY OF FAITH IN YOUR HEART.

I believe that if you took the time to purchase this book there was something tugging at your Spirit telling you that you needed to read it. And if that is the case, then

I imagine there is an area in your life that you need to improve on and most likely it is stemming from a disbelief that you can't get better. Or someone has told you "there are no options". Don't believe this. There are always options. I always find options for my patients or the options find me. Maybe not in the way I would expect, but an answer always shows up because my patients and I believe!

This book is designed to lay a groundwork in understanding:

1. How the body works;

2. How diseases come about if something is wrong with #1;

3. What treatment options you can choose from (Conventional, Alternative, or Naturopathic); and

4. How the **Power of Belief** affects outcomes in health. Conventional Medicine is designed to treat or manage symptoms using medications or surgeries, Alternative Medicine provides "natural" means for symptom management, and Naturopathic Medicine focuses on treating causes.

Treating causes of diseases forces the practitioner to maintain a patient-centered practice, as every cause will be different for every patient even if they share symptoms. Regardless, each system of medicine is needed. I maintain the belief that eventually there will be a more graceful flow between the systems of medicine, as there is a time and place for each.

Dr. Brandie Gowey, NMD
www.goweyresearchgroup.com

Part I

Biochemistry 101

Most diseases can be traced to a malfunction-ing of processes within or between the cells of our bodies. In this section, I will describe some of the most basic functions our cells perform. If something "goes astray" with one or more of these functions disease can manifest.

Knowing where something has "gone wrong" with a cell becomes part of treating causes.

❧ 1 ❧
Cell-to-Cell
Communication

Your cells have outer membranes built like fences: the "fences" are constructed with row upon row of fats and proteins (www.en.wikipedia.org/wiki/Cell_membrane). These "fences" have very important functions. First, they allow cells to communicate with one another. Second, they regulate movement of proteins, minerals, vitamins, and hormones from the blood to the inside of the cell, and vice versa. See Figure 1.

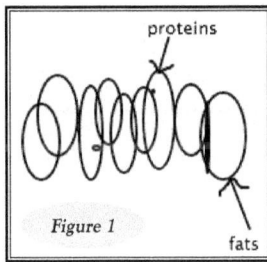

Figure 1.

Very simplistic drawing of a cell membrane made up of fats (lipids) and protein (author's rendition of a cell membrane, adapted from Guyton and Hall 2000).

This membrane is so important that Dr. Michael Murray, ND and Jade Reutler R.R.T, R.C.P, state it as such:

> *The basic function of the cell membrane is to serve as a selective barrier that regulates the passage of certain material in and out of the cell…with a disturbance in cellular membrane structure or function, there is a disruption of virtually all cellular processes (Murray and Reutler 1996).*

Ideally, the cell membrane "fences" are composed of protein (from foods such as meats or nuts) and fats called "Omega oils" (such as Omega 3, 6, and 9). Omega 3s are found in fish and plant oils, Omega 6 in vegetable oils, and Omega 9 in olive oil. The right balance of Omega oils in our diet gives us healthy cell membranes, keeping our energy levels good and inflammation in check.

The American diet tends to have too little Omega oils. Because of this, cell membranes aren't as healthy, cell-to-cell communication decreases, energy levels drop, and inflammation starts. To complicate the situation more, some Omega oils (the Omega 6s) promote inflammation if their levels are excessively higher than the Omega 3s. Ideally, we need to consume about 4:1 ratio of Omega 6:3. With the amount of veggie oils we currently consume, most Americans get 20:1 Omega 6:3 in their diets (Murray and Reutler 1996). Veggie oils are grossly classed as corn, canola, and soy.

Omega oils aren't the only types of fats we consume. We also eat saturated fats (in animal fats) and manufactured fats called trans, hydrogenated, or partially hydroge-nated. All of these fats may contribute to the development of inflammation if they are in excess in the diet. Trans fats, hydrogenated oils, and partially hydrogenated oils interrupt cell-to-cell communication (my theory). Trans/hydrogenated/partially hy-drogenated fats are not made in nature. They are oils manipulated by technology such that they can keep for months on store shelves without going bad. See Figures 2 and 3.

Figure 2. ☞

This diagram demonstrates fat metabolism and how the different fats either promote or diminish health. This is a drawing I did for a patient on 12/19/12, adapted from information in Dr. Murray's book, Understanding Fats and Oils.

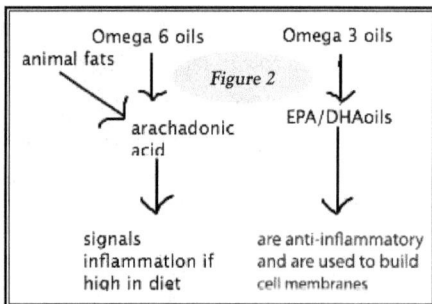

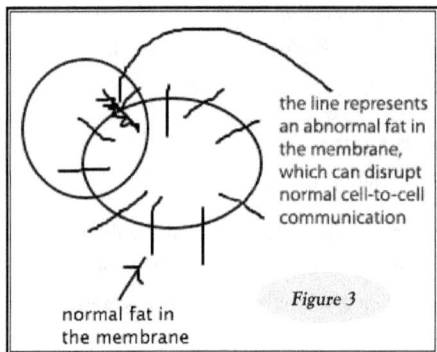

Omega 6 oils	Omega 3 oils
animal fats	

Figure 2

arachadonic acid

EPA/DHAoils

signals inflammation if high in diet

are anti-inflammatory and are used to build cell membranes

the line represents an abnormal fat in the membrane, which can disrupt normal cell-to-cell communication

normal fat in the membrane

Figure 3

☞ Figure 3.

My idea of what a trans-fat (hydrogenated or partially hydrogenated) in the cell membrane looks like. Cells can't communicate if their membranes aren't healthy.

If you consistently consume high amounts of Omega 6 oils as well as trans/hydroge-nated/partially hydrogenated fats, your cell-to-cell communication will not be healthy. In my clinical experience, many diseases result from too many trans and hydrogenated oils, and too low Omega 3 oils.

Examples of Diseases include:

Abnormal Heart Rhythms	Autism (Lyall et al. 2013)	Depression
Anxiety	Autoimmune Diseases	Diabetes
Atherosclerosis	Cancer	Heart Disease

Saturated fats also get a bad rap, but I think they are only "bad" if the animal the fats came from was full of hormones, chemicals, or antibiotics. Some saturated fat is good because it is such an excellent energy source.

✌ 2 ✌
Harnessing Energy from Food

With a healthy cell membrane of good fats and protein (Chapter 1), your body is ready to obtain energy from the foods you eat. This process requires several steps and ultimately produces an energy molecule called ATP (adenosine triphosphate).

It is easier for me to explain this transformative process with drawings. Therefore, this chapter is a series of figures (Figures 4-6) simplified from drawings I created to tutor classmates while I was in medical school. Key steps, vitamins, and minerals are highlighted (Champe and Harvey 1994).

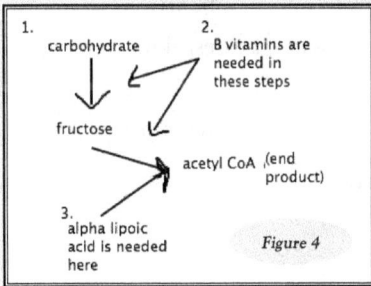

Figure 4.

This is the first step in harnessing energy (ATP) from food, called glycolysis.

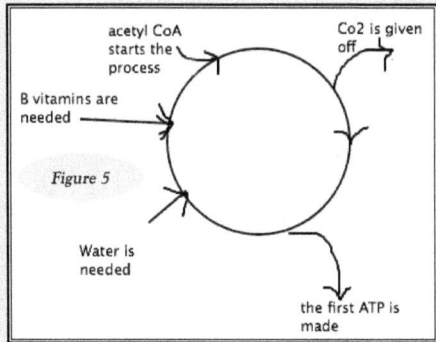

Figure 5.

This is the second step in harnessing energy (ATP) from food, called the Krebs or TCA cycle.

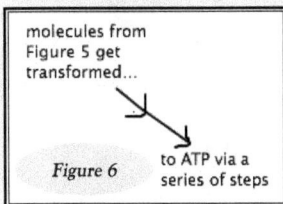

Figure 6.

The last step in harnessing energy (ATP) from food, called the Electron Transport System (ETS). Most of our energy is produced at this step (Chapter 3).

In my clinical experience, problems in any of these pathways (Figures 4-6) inhibits the ability of our cells to obtain energy from food, allowing for the development of Chronic Diseases such as:

Adrenal Fatigue

Anxiety

Asthma/Lung Disorders

Arthritis

Cancer

Chronic Colds/Flu

Chronic Ear Infections

Chronic Fatigue Syndrome

Chronic Sinus Infections

Degenerative Diseases of the Spine

Depression

Eczema

Gallbladder

Problems/Diseases

Fibromyalgia

Heart Disease

Hormone Disorders

Irritable Bowel Disease

Low Libido

Memory Loss

Menstrual Difficulties

Neurological Diseases

Obesity

Skin Diseases/Skin Cancer

Sleep Disorders

Thyroid Dysfunction

Any disease, really…

❧ 3 ❧
Harnessing Energy from Food:
The Final & Most Important Piece

In the previous chapter, I presented the various steps required to harness energy from foods. The final step (shown in Figure 6) is performed by a tiny part within the cell called the mitochondria.

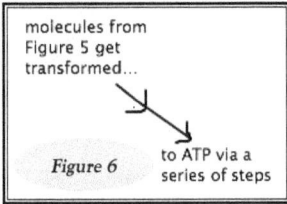

molecules from Figure 5 get transformed...

Figure 6 — to ATP via a series of steps

☜ *Figure 6.*

The last step in harnessing energy (ATP) from food, called the Electron Transport System (ETS). Most of our energy is produced at this step (Chapter 2).

The Mitochondria require a great deal of Nutrients to perform their work.
Below is a summary of the Nutrients they require (Crinnion 2003-4):

B Vitamins	Alpha Lipoic Acid	Trace Minerals
Magnesium	Vitamin C	Water
L-carnitine	Manganese	Oxygen

Mitochondrial function deteriorates with changes in nutrient levels, environmental toxins, and inflammation (Lopez-Armada et al. 2012). I can test mitochondria activity levels by measuring the activity level of an enzyme called "superoxide dismutase". Superoxide dismutase regulates mitochondrial activity. I have found that both over and under activity of mitochondrial superoxide dismutase is indicative of disease processes (Figure 7).

Protection *Figure 7*			Reference Range
★ Glutathione	786		>= 669 micromol/L
Total Antioxidant Capacity (TAC)	0.61		>= 0.54 mmol/L
Cysteine		0.68	0.46-1.20 mg/dL
Sulphate	3.0		3.0-5.9 mg/dL
Cysteine/Sulphate		0.23	0.12-0.32
Cystine		2.23	1.60-3.20 mg/dL
Cysteine/Cystine Ratio		0.30	0.17-0.50
Enzymes			**Reference Range**
★ Glutathione Peroxidase		32.1	20.0-38.0 U/g Hb
Superoxide Dismutase		22,674	5,275-16,662 U/g Hb

Figure 7. Mitochondrial function is shown by the activity of superoxide dismutase, a key enzyme measurable via blood work. This is an example of mitochondrial activity from a patient with heart disease.

**In my clinical experience, diseases that may manifest
due to impaired Mitochondrial Function include:**

Amyotrophic Lateral Sclerosis
(ALS)

Anxiety

Arthritis

Asthma/Lung Diseases

Chronic Fatigue

Depression

Diabetes

Fibromyalgia

Heart Disease

Menieres Disease

Multiple Sclerosis (MS)

Thyroid Dysfunction

Tinnitus

Weight Change

❧ 4 ❧
Detoxification Pathways: Glutathione & Cytochrome P450

Every moment that we are alive our body is working to eliminate toxins. Patients always look at me like they are surprised when I say this, but it is true: at any given moment your body is processing things like mercury in auto exhaust, vaccines, solvent odors in cleaners, fumes from building supplies, pesticides in food, medications, or supplements (just to name a few). Anything that our body does not make could be classed as a "toxin" because it is something foreign to our natural, inherent processes and therefore is something our body works to eliminate.

There are many pathways and processes by which this toxin elimination occurs. In my opinion, the two most important are glutathione and Cytochrome P450.

Glutathione is a molecule like pieces to a puzzle. These puzzle pieces are composed of amino acids (which come from protein) and Vitamin C (Waters 2003-4). The glue holding the puzzle pieces together involves the use of hydrogen. When a toxin comes in contact with glutathione, it (the glutathione) gives the hydrogen to the toxin. This binding aids in the toxin elimination (Figure 8).

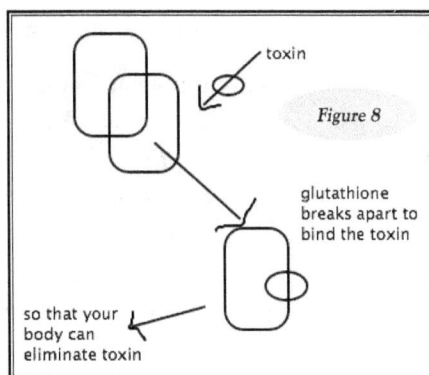

toxin

Figure 8

glutathione breaks apart to bind the toxin

so that your body can eliminate toxin

Figure 8. 🖝

Glutathione
(www.en.wikipedia.org/wiki/Glutathione).

If glutathione levels are low, toxins will continue to circulate in the bloodstream, potentially creating an inflammatory reaction. This reaction damages body tissues and organs (Crinnion 2003-4 and my clinical experience). You can test for low glutathione levels via a precursor in the blood called "homocysteine" (Lord and Fitzgerald 2006) or you can use the specialty lab Genova Diagnostics to directly test levels.

Research from Soto et al. (1998) shows that blood levels of glutathione may be normal, while gut tissue levels aren't. This means body demand is different in different tissues. There are supplemental forms of glutathione on the market, but I am not convinced they absorb well; my patients on oral glutathione never noticed a difference in their symptoms until I switched them to a different mode of administration (IV, intramuscular, or sublingual). Sublingual is a form I created and is available on How-DoITreatNaturally.com.

I have found that patients metabolize glutathione in unpredictable ways. Some do very well on it while others see adverse effects. Here are examples:

- Patient with high estrogen levels started on a 1 cc glutathione injection (IM) but gained weight; we lowered the dose and she started to lose weight.
- Patient gaining weight from a hormone IUD (Meriva) was able to lose weight on 1 cc (IM) of 200 mg weekly without any problems.
- Patient diagnosed as being bipolar can only do glutathione at 0.5 mg via IV; higher doses cause insomnia but 0.5 mg makes her feel "great".
- MS patient has no muscle spasms with 600 mg glutathione via IV.
- Patient with painful menstrual cramps experiences a decrease in pain after 0.5 cc (IM) glutathione.

Be careful if you choose to go on glutathione and work with your physician on mode of administration. Start with low doses if you are going to do IV or IM glutathione. Or you can start with the sublingual and work your way into trying it IV/IM.

Cytochrome enzyme system: These are groupings of enzymes highly concentrated in your liver, lungs, and gut (Waters 2003-4). Researchers have identified what are "normal" groupings of these enzymes, but many of us have changes from these "normals" called "polymorphisms". For example, if you struggle with side effects from medications you take, you may have a deficiency in your Cytochrome system (perhaps the "polymorphism"). You can test to see what Cytochrome enzymes you are low in via the company Genova Diagnostics (Figure 9).

PHASE I Detoxification: The First Line of Defense

Figure 9

In Phase I detoxification, enzymes, known collectively as the cytochrome P-450 system, use oxygen to modify toxic compounds, drugs, or steroid hormones. Many toxins must undergo Phase II detoxification after a reactive site has been formed. Because there are many different toxic compounds the body might encounter, there are many variants of Phase I enzymes.

	Cytochrome P-450		
Result	Gene	internet information	
✔	CYP1A1	www.genovations.com/gdgen01	
●	CYP1B1	www.genovations.com/gdgen02	
✔	CYP2A6	www.genovations.com/gdgen10	
●	CYP2C9	www.genovations.com/gdgen05	
✔	CYP2C19	www.genovations.com/gdgen06	
✔	CYP2D6	www.genovations.com/gdgen03	
✔	CYP2E1	www.genovations.com/gdgen04	
✔	CYP3A4	www.genovations.com/gdgen07	

● = positive

Your Results: Polymorphisms (SNPs) in the genes coding for a particular enzyme can increase or, more commonly, decrease the activity of that enzyme. Both increased and decreased activity may be harmful. Increased phase I clearance without increased clearance in Phase II can lead to the formation of toxic intermediates that may be more toxic than the original toxin. Decreased Phase I clearance will cause toxic accumulation in the body. Adverse reactions to drugs are often due to a decreased capacity for clearing them from the system.

Figure 9. This is an example test done on a patient via Genova Diagnostics of common cytochrome levels/pathways.

In my clinical experience, the following diseases may manifest from Low Glutathione and/or Cytochrome P450 Systems:

Arthritis

Asthma

Cancer

Cervical Dysplasia

Chronic Fatigue

Chronic Obstructive
Pulmonary Disease (COPD)

Depression/Anxiety

Drug Sensitivity

Emphysema

Fatty Liver

Fibromyalgia

Headaches

Heart Disease

Hormonal Diseases/Problems

Insomnia

Irritable Bowel Syndrome (IBS)

Macular Degeneration

Odor/Pollution Sensitivity

Painful Menses

Symptomatic Menopause

Sensitivity to Supplements/
Herbal Medicines

❦ 5 ❦
Detoxification:
Antioxidants and Apoptosis

Ten or so years ago, the importance of quenching "free radicals" hit the supplement market (www.healthchecksystems.com/antioxid.htm). I took for granted what anti-oxidants were until I started working with patients who were struggling with abnormal Pap smears (cervical dysplasia): the probability of shifting the dysplasia (which is pre-cancer) to normal increased when I recommended the patients add high-dose antioxidants to their diet.

Antioxidants are the color-rich pigments in plants (in fruits and veggies), such as the orange in carrots, the blue in blueberries, the red in raspberries. These colors help induce a process called "apoptosis". Apoptosis is the process within your cells that recognizes when a cell's DNA has been damaged and signals it to die off so a new one can come in to replace it.

No Plant Pigments = Limited Apoptosis

(www.en.wikipedia.org/wiki/Antioxidant).
Without apoptosis, damaged cells stay damaged.

**In my clinical experience, the following diseases
are linked to Low Antioxidant, Low Apoptotic processes:**

Cancer	Fatty Liver
Skin Sancer	KidneyDiseases
Pre-cancerous Conditions (such as Cervical Dysplasia)	Macular Degeneration
Fibromyalgia	Glaucoma
Heart Disease	Diabetes
Skin Diseases	Lung Diseases
	Any Disease, really…

❧ 6 ❧
The Immune System

I tell patients the immune system is like a table full of ping-pong balls. The ping-pong balls are all nicely arranged on the table until something causes them to start moving. Imagine someone throwing one ping-pong ball (a trigger) at this table of ping-pong balls, and all of the chaos and movement that would happen once that one ping-pong ball is thrown—that's how your immune system can operate. Triggers to the ping-pong ball immune system include damaged cells, viruses, bacteria, toxins, or other immune cells (Horseen et al. 2012).

The Immune System is Composed of Two Types of "Ping-Pong" Balls (Cells):

Signaling Molecules (Proteins)   White Blood Cells

Subdivided further, White Blood Cells include:

Basophils   Monocytes (Macrophages)

Eosinophils   Neutrophils

Lymphocytes (B and T cells)

Signaling Molecules (Proteins) include:

Cytokines   Interleukins

Glial Cells   Prostaglandins

Signaling molecules are communicators within the ping-pong ball system, and I liken them to the Internet: they communicate to other immune cells that something is going on.

The triggering process within the immune system is both blessing and curse. A little bit of triggering is good. For example, if you were recently exposed to a virus or bacteria, you need your white blood cells to start working to combat the infection. But if the infection goes on for too long you may start to experience tissue damage. Technically, this process is called inflammation (Figure 10), which is fed by signaling molecules.

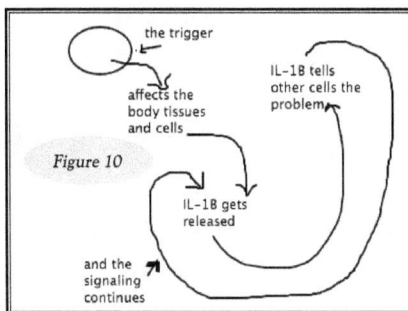

Figure 10. ☞

Example of how the immune system signals inflammation (as shown by IL-1B, a type of interleukin).

Some signaling molecules (such as interleukins) can be tested with the specialty lab company Genova Diagnostics. The signaling molecule called IL-1B is the one that causes a lot of problems for patients dealing with chronic pain as from arthritis (Eder 2009). Figure 11 shows IL-1B levels in a patient with very advanced osteoarthritis.

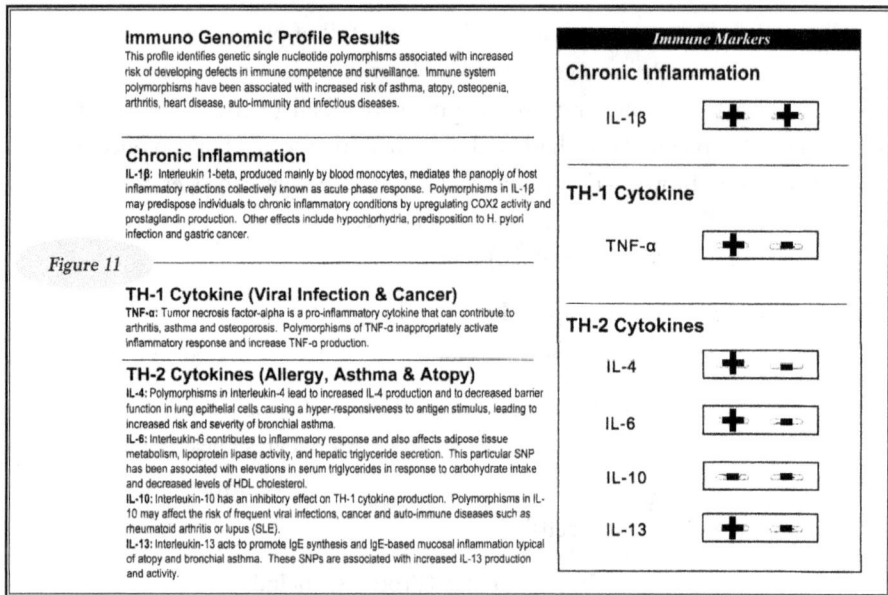

Figure 11

Immuno Genomic Profile Results
This profile identifies genetic single nucleotide polymorphisms associated with increased risk of developing defects in immune competence and surveillance. Immune system polymorphisms have been associated with increased risk of asthma, atopy, osteopenia, arthritis, heart disease, auto-immunity and infectious diseases.

Chronic Inflammation
IL-1β: Interleukin 1-beta, produced mainly by blood monocytes, mediates the panoply of host inflammatory reactions collectively known as acute phase response. Polymorphisms in IL-1β may predispose individuals to chronic inflammatory conditions by upregulating COX2 activity and prostaglandin production. Other effects include hypochlorhydria, predisposition to H. pylori infection and gastric cancer.

TH-1 Cytokine (Viral Infection & Cancer)
TNF-α: Tumor necrosis factor-alpha is a pro-inflammatory cytokine that can contribute to arthritis, asthma and osteoporosis. Polymorphisms of TNF-α inappropriately activate inflammatory response and increase TNF-α production.

TH-2 Cytokines (Allergy, Asthma & Atopy)
IL-4: Polymorphisms in interleukin-4 lead to increased IL-4 production and to decreased barrier function in lung epithelial cells causing a hyper-responsiveness to antigen stimulus, leading to increased risk and severity of bronchial asthma.
IL-6: Interleukin-6 contributes to inflammatory response and also affects adipose tissue metabolism, lipoprotein lipase activity, and hepatic triglyceride secretion. This particular SNP has been associated with elevations in serum triglycerides in response to carbohydrate intake and decreased levels of HDL cholesterol.
IL-10: Interleukin-10 has an inhibitory effect on TH-1 cytokine production. Polymorphisms in IL-10 may affect the risk of frequent viral infections, cancer and auto-immune diseases such as rheumatoid arthritis or lupus (SLE).
IL-13: Interleukin-13 acts to promote IgE synthesis and IgE-based mucosal inflammation typical of atopy and bronchial asthma. These SNPs are associated with increased IL-13 production and activity.

Immune Markers

Chronic Inflammation

IL-1β

TH-1 Cytokine

TNF-α

TH-2 Cytokines

IL-4

IL-6

IL-10

IL-13

Figure 11. Genova-Diagnostics test showing expression of IL-1B.

In my clinical experience, I have seen the following diseases manifest because of Systemic Inflammation:

Allergies

Asthma

Autoimmune Diseases

Cancer

Celiac Disease

Cellulitis/Other Infections

Chronic Pain

Degeneration of Spine/Stenosis

Depression

Early Aging

Eczema

Fatigue

Fibromyalgia

Glaucoma/Macular Degeneration

Headaches

Heart Disease

IBS

Kidney Diseases

Liver Diseases

MS/Other Neurological Diseases

Osteoarthritis

Rheumatoid Arthritis

༒ 7 ༒
The Nervous System

Just like your immune system, your nervous system is extremely complex. The nervous system helps us move, feel sensations, and experience emotion. Neurotransmitters are the primary molecules that are active in this system; they function within nerves and help communicate the experiences such as movement, temperature, touch, emotion, or pain.

Neurotransmitters are primarily made from protein, Vitamin C, magnesium, and B vitamins. Below is a very basic schematic of neurotransmitter production and function.

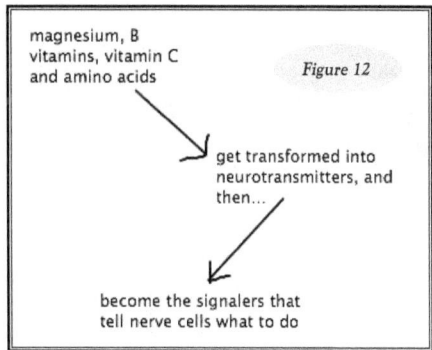

```
magnesium, B
vitamins, vitamin C
and amino acids                        Figure 12


                          get transformed into
                          neurotransmitters, and
                          then...


                  become the signalers that
                  tell nerve cells what to do
```

Figure 12. ☞

The making of a neurotransmitter
(Guyton and Hall 2000).

Once a neurotransmitter is made by a nervous system cell, it gets released into the space adjoining a nearby cell and acts like a phone signal: the signal continues to other cells until the message is fully conveyed for an end result (such as moving your arm or experiencing an emotion).

**Diseases that may manifest from Low Neurotransmitter Levels,
High Neurotransmitter Levels, or Nerve Damage include:**

Anxiety	Heart Arrhythmias
Back Pain	IBS
Depression	MS
Fibromyalgia	Radiculopathy

ᘒ 8 ᘒ

Hormones

Hormones are tiny molecules that regulate body functions such as blood sugar levels, mood, menstruation, libido, blood pressure, weight, metabolism, or immune system function. Hormones are made by glands such as the pituitary, testes, pineal, thyroid, adrenals, or ovaries.

In my practice, I see most problems in terms of symptoms and diseases coming from the thyroid and adrenal glands. The thyroid produces T4 (and some T3). T4 is made of iodine and the amino acid tyrosine; once it gets made it is released into the bloodstream where it is converted in the presence of selenium and zinc into T3. T3 is the hormone that is brought into the cells and is metabolically active (Greenspan and Strewler 1997).

The adrenals take cholesterol, Vitamin D, Vitamin C, magnesium, and B vitamins to make hormones such as estrogen, testosterone, progesterone, DHEA, and cortisol (Waters 2003-4).

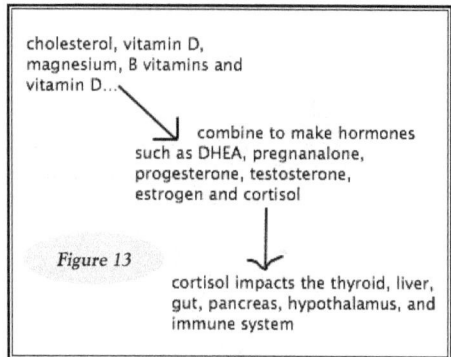

Figure 13. 🖘
The flow and production of hormones from the thyroid and adrenal glands.
(Gowey 2014).

cholesterol, vitamin D,
magnesium, B vitamins and
vitamin D...

combine to make hormones
such as DHEA, pregnanalone,
progesterone, testosterone,
estrogen and cortisol

Figure 13

cortisol impacts the thyroid, liver,
gut, pancreas, hypothalamus, and
immune system

Thyroid Hormone Helps Regulate:

Energy Levels	Metabolism	Temperature
Hair/Skin/Nails	Mood	Weight

Adrenal Hormones Help Regulate:

Age of Menarche	Feelings of Restfulness	Sleep/Wake Cycle
Appetite	Immune System	Thyroid
Blood Pressure	Libido	Weight
Blood Sugars	Menstrual Cycles	Weight Gain/Loss
Bone Density	Metabolism	(especially
Drive	Mood	Abdominal Weight)
Energy Levels	Muscle Mass	

Of all the hormones produced by the adrenals, the one I help patients with the most is cortisol (Figure 14). Cortisol has a daily rhythm: normally it is elevated in the morning which helps you wake up, has a few peaks and valleys throughout the day, and then lowers at night helping you sleep. This cycle keeps your blood sugar normal (even when you're not eating), keeps your mood stable, keeps blood pressure normal, and your immune system healthy. Figure 14 is an example of a normal cortisol rhythm.

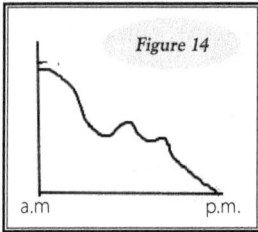

Figure 14.

The normal cortisol cycle (adopted from an adrenal stress test by DiagnosTechs).

Adrenal cortisol is extremely sensitive to stress. Any kind of stressor can affect the cortisol cycle. Acute stress increases cortisol levels; chronic stress may increase or decrease cortisol. Regardless of the length of time of the stress or type of stress, when cortisol levels change you will experience symptoms.

**Examples of Various Cortisol Levels
and the Symptoms that May Manifest as a Result**

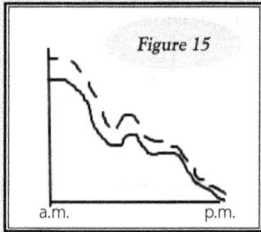

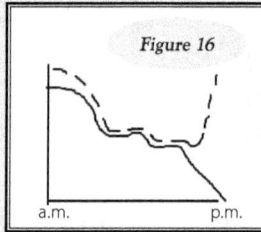

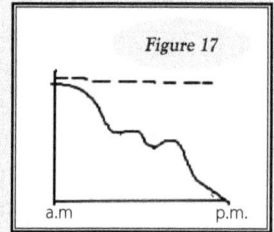

Figure 15.

Figure 16.

Figure 17.

Elevated cortisol in the morning causes early waking. The solid line indicates normal cortisol rhythm.

Elevated cortisol at night causes insomnia. The solid line indicates normal cortisol rhythm.

Elevated cortisol during the day can cause high blood sugar levels, weight gain, changes in blood pressure, or frequent colds. The solid line indicates normal cortisol rhythm.

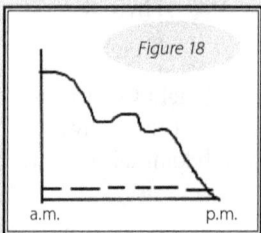

Figure 18.

Low a.m. or day cortisol levels lead to feelings of depression or anxiety, weight changes, memory loss, and inattention. The solid line indicates normal cortisol rhythm.

When I first started practicing medicine, I would order a test of cortisol levels on patients I suspected were struggling with their adrenal function. The best test to use is a saliva test, not blood work. Blood work is not sensitive enough and will only pick up on very dramatic changes in cortisol. However, I don't actually use the saliva test anymore as I can tell when patients are struggling with the adrenals (based on their symptoms).

Even though I focus a lot on the adrenals, any hormone imbalance can create adverse symptoms.

Examples of diseases that manifest from changes to Hormone Levels:

ADHD	Depression
Anxiety	Diabetes
Arthritis	Fibromyalgia
Autoimmune Diseases	Goiters
Bipolar/Other Mental/Emotional Diseases	Heart Palpitations
Cancer	Hormone Levels Changes/Diseases
Cardiovascular Disease	Insomnia
Chronic Fatigue	Painful Menstrual Cramps

❧ 9 ❧
The Internal Master

I encourage all my patients to follow their heart. We all have potential; something we are either good at or something we can do well for the benefit of others. The longer I practice medicine the more I see the link between disease and NOT following the potential we feel in our hearts: without the manifestation of our potential, disease may show instead (clinical observation and Jarrett 2000).

According to Eastern Philosophy (rooted in Taoism, which is the core of acupuncture), we all have a "destiny" to manifest (Jarrett 2000). This "destiny" or inner potential is imparted to us spiritually at the moment of conception, and is nourished—or not nourished—as we grow up. This potential is housed energetically by different parts of our anatomy, and the connections between the various aspects of our anatomy work together to help us bring forth our potential. This philosophy states that manifestation of potential is only something that happens if that is something already within us.

For example, everyone wants to be financially well off. But maybe that kind of wealth is not in your spiritual DNA: maybe your abundance comes from somewhere or something else. If you try to "manifest" wealth and you are NOT working with what you feel in your heart to do, think, or say, then financial abundance will not come to you. If in your heart you feel you are meant to own your own business and instead you are working at a job you dislike, how do you think wealth will come to you? What would happen if you listened to your heart and tapped into the inner abundance? Would the right abundance for you then manifest? The key is persisting with following what is in your heart and not giving up until the right conditions help you bring things forth. This may take several years: this is not an overnight process and I say this from experience!

> By acknowledging and nourishing what has been placed within, and accepting all situations in life as opportunities for self-cultivation, the sage manifests destiny...the appropriate use of the mind is as a tool for self-discovery and as the commander of the qi, which allows us to take actions in the world consistent with the intentions in our heart...instead of causing pain and generating illness over life's ups and downs, the sage goes along with what has been allotted...(Jarrett 2000).

ANY disease can manifest if we are not working toward bringing forth our potential.

Part II

The "Diseases"

In Part I, we discuss basic biochemical pathways of the body. In Part II, we are going to look at the most common diseases—their diagnosis, symptoms, and causes underlying their manifestation.

Most diseases will resolve once you work to identify and treat the cause unless they are exclusively genetically or congenitally linked. But even if you have a disease that is more difficult to treat such as osteoarthritis or cancer, understanding the cause of the arthritis or cancer can prevent it from becoming worse or help guide you in better treatment options.

In this section, I will also help you understand the differences in the various systems of medicine. Currently we have three dominant forms of medicine to choose from: Conventional, Alternative, and Naturopathic.

✛ **Conventional Medicine** is the main form of medicine we have today (MDs or DOs practice this kind of medicine). It focuses on treating symptoms with medications or surgeries.

✳ **Alternative Medicine** uses natural substances to treat symptoms.

✪ **Naturopathic Medicine** treats causes and may use a natural substance or medication to do so.

I do not classify Naturopathic Medicine in Alternative Medicine because "alternative" implies use of a substance or modality in place of a Conventionally prescribed medication. Naturopathic Medicine first establishes the cause(s), then develops a treatment plan based on the cause(s), fitting that plan to the individual. Naturopathic Medical Doctors may use an "alternative" modality to treat the cause or they may prescribe a medication. Some providers are now using the term "Integrative" to describe a practice that is a blend of Conventional Medicine and Alternative or Naturopathic. I find this term to be very confusing, as both Conventional and Naturopathic Physicians use it. To really understand the philosophical perspective from which your doctor practices, you will have to do some investigating to discover their approach. A good Naturopathic-minded Doctor will always work to identify the cause before they develop any kind of treatment plan for you, regardless of whether or not they call themselves "Integrative" or "Alternative".

It is important to know the differences in the paradigms of medicine so that you know when you will need each. For example, if you have a sudden onset of abdominal pain you will want to go to the emergency room. But if all your results return as "normal" you may want to call your Naturopathic Physician to identify a deeper cause.

Acupuncture, homeopathy, herbal medicine, and massage are treatment modalities that could be classed as Alternative or Naturopathic. These are medicines that can be used either to address symptoms or deeper causes.

❧ 10 ☙
Chronic Cold/Flu

The common cold or flu is triggered by a virus. The virus stimulates symptoms such as cough, fever, body aches, fatigue, muscle pain, or diarrhea. These symptoms result from your immune system sending out signaling molecules (Chapter 6) in response to the presence of the virus.

Influenza is Diagnosed via:
Physical Exam and History

✚ Conventional Medical Treatment Options include:
Flu Vaccine
Antibiotics
Fluids
Over-the-counter Medications

Of the treatments listed above, Conventional Medicine considers the flu vaccine the "most important aspect of prevention" (www.mdconsult.com/das/pdxmd/body/404981776-3/0?type=med&eid=9-u1.0-_1_mt_1014549).

✻ Alternative Medical Treatment Options include:
Herbs
Fluids
Vitamins
Homeopathic Medicines

✪ Naturopathic Medicine, Treating the Cause:

If your immune system is strong you generally won't get the flu, even if your body is exposed to the virus that "causes" the flu. I think the flu, like any other virus, is only a problem if our system is weak: if the immune system isn't strong, then the virus will become very active and create symptoms.

Commonly, flu symptoms come from a problem with the gut: the gut houses most of our immune cells and I have noticed a correlation between those suffering from the flu and gut disorders.

Here is a case to illustrate my point:

A 73-year-old patient struggled with extensive bouts of the flu, bronchitis, and/or pneumonia every year since she was a young girl. Her history included irritable bowel syndrome, fibromyalgia, colitis, and kidney problems including symptoms such as bloating, abdominal pain, diarrhea, or constipation.

I started working with her by ordering a food sensitivity test. Food sensitivities can create inflammation and ultimately lead to many of the diseases and conditions she chronically suffered from.

Here is a list of foods she was sensitive to:

Amaranth	Cumin	Oat
Broccoli	Egg	Papaya
Cauliflower	Ginger	Pineapple
Crab	Milk (Cow)	Pumpkin
Cranberry	Mushrooms	Wheat

I had her eliminate these foods as best she could. After a few weeks of avoiding them (especially eggs, dairy, and wheat) most of the abdominal pain was gone. She still had gas, bloating, constipation, and diarrhea, so I added a light dose of probiotics. These reduced both constipation and diarrhea. After that, I added a rectal suppository of glutathione (100 mg) that I had Tenille Davis (pharmacist) at Civic Center Pharmacy formulate for me. Research is showing links between low gut glutathione levels and abdominal diseases (Soto et al. 1998). I wanted to ensure the glutathione would absorb locally so I had the pharmacist make a rectal formulation. This treatment protocol eliminated all of her abdominal symptoms.

The year we started this treatment was the first time since childhood she did not get pneumonia, bronchitis, or even the cold/flu over the winter. She has been flu-free since.

Your gut has collections of white blood cells responsible for responding to viruses, bacteria, and inflammation. Food sensitivities create inflammation. Most of your immune cells are in your gut. If your immune system is preoccupied dealing with inflammation from food sensitivities, it is more difficult to fight off a viral or bacterial infection (clinical experience). Dairy, wheat, eggs, beans, nuts, bananas, sugar, cranberries, and GMO (genetically modified) foods are very common culprits of gut inflammation. I often have patients start with limiting these foods when I am working with them to heal their intestinal tract.

Stress is also a contributing factor to coming down with a cold or flu. Stress increases the output of the hormone cortisol (Chapter 8). When cortisol increases, it actually has an effect of suppressing the immune system. Then when you get exposed to a bug, you will get sick easier and most likely for a longer period of time than someone who is not stressed. I support my patients who are in this position by getting them on a good adrenal boosting program, such as use of my adrenal herbs (see my website) or a good vitamin IV infusion. High dose vitamins, especially Vitamin C, support the adrenals ability to make hormones.

Treating the Cause with the Power of Belief:

My patients know their bodies. After working with me for a while, I hear patients who used to say things like, "I don't know why I got sick, must be the bad flu this year and I didn't get my flu shot", to "I was super stressed out recently and eating bad and I got sick and I know that is why I got sick and can I please get a Vitamin C IV?"

When you start to get to know your body, you automatically believe you can get well by giving it what it needs. It becomes an unconscious expression of your conscience: you know what you need even if you start to get sick because you have tapped into a belief that you do not have to be unhealthy or live in fear that you may become sick. If you get sick, you deal with it, gracefully.

Here is what I have taught my patients to do if they start to get an Illness:

1. Identify the cause; more often than not it is stress or poor diet choices that start the illness.

2. Rest.

3. Take immune supportive herbs, such as Astragalus.

4. Avoid processed sugars (Chapter 15).

5. Eat lightly (broth and steamed veggies are great).

6. Journal.

7. Take time out for you.

❧ 11 ❧
Common Illnesses in Children

Children have very delicate immune systems. They are not born with the level of immune function adults have; therefore, they tend to get sick more often. In my clinical experience, I see it can take several years from birth for a healthy immune system to develop. Children start to build their immune system from the white blood cells (Chapter 6) in breast milk.

Illnesses in Children are Usually Diagnosed via:
Symptom Presentation
Physical Exam

✚ Conventional Medical Treatment Options include:
Laxatives (for Constipation)
Antibiotics (for Ear Infections)
Corticosteroid Oral or as Breathing Treatment (for Asthma)
Topical Corticosteroids (for Eczema)

✳ Alternative Medical Treatment Options include:
Herbs
Supplements such as Probiotics
Homeopathic Medicines
Humidifiers with Essential Oils

❂ Naturopathic Medicine, Treating the Cause:
In my opinion, food sensitivities are a significant cause of illnesses in kids because they create inflammation. This inflammation impacts the white blood cells and stimulates the activity of signaling molecules (the ping-pong balls/Internet signal, Chapter 6). For my patients, I start with having mom (or caregivers) eliminate cow dairy from the child's diet (if the mom is breastfeeding, she needs to eliminate cow dairy as well because the cow milk proteins will get into her milk). This includes most formulas and cow's milk yogurt.

While the child is coming off Dairy, I recommend:
Probiotics
DHA/EPA or Fish Oils
Liquid Multivitamin/Mineral

Integrative Therapeutics V-clear Homeopathic
(helps boost the immune system's response to viruses safely)

Immune Supportive Herbs (i.e. Astragalus or Elderberry)

If cow dairy is NOT the cause of the symptoms, other foods may be culprits, such as wheat. I may recommend a food sensitivity panel at this time to help us identify foods we may be missing. Children can also be sensitive to GMO (genetically modified) foods or non-organic ones: if the child has a sensitivity to the chemicals in the food or the genetic modification of it, the food will not as likely show up on a food test. In other words, if it doesn't show up but the child is still reacting, it may then mean the chemicals, hormones, or genetic modification of the food is what the child is sensitive to. Either way, the food needs to be eliminated as best as possible.

**Here is a Milk Formula I provide to parents
as an alternative to cow's milk products on the market:**

- 4-5 cups goat, soy, or rice milk (organic, hormone-free, and GMO-free preferably)

- Drop probiotics (liquid or open a capsule and put contents in)

- ½-1 tsp Nordic Naturals Omega oils for kids

- Dose of a liquid multivitamin and fat-soluble vitamins such as A/D/E

You can make this in large batches and keep it in the fridge or freezer for later. This formula has the Omega oils and supportive nutrients your child will need to build healthy digestive and immune systems.

A friend of mine took dairy out of her nine-month-old's diet per my recommendation and a few weeks later we were both amazed by the changes. Prior to a dairy free diet, the child had fused labia, constipation, abdominal pains, and was not talking. After going dairy-free, the labia actually separated and the child became very animated. Abdominal discomforts also resolved.

You never know how much little things can or will make a difference.

Here are the most Common Illnesses in Children and Common Causes of each Disease:

Colic: *Cow Dairy or Wheat*

Constipation: *Cow Dairy*

Eczema: *Any Food (do a food sensitivity test) or Low Probiotic Levels*

Ear Infections: *Cow Dairy*

Asthma: *Cow Dairy or Wheat, Stress/Anxiety*

Gut Pains: *Any Food (Cow Dairy and Eggs are the most common)*

Behavioral Challenges: *Sugar*

Insomnia, Frequent Waking: *Sugar*

Treating the Cause with the Power of Belief:

My friend, who had taken her daughter off dairy, is a Speech Pathologist specializing in Social Thinking. She works with children diagnosed with conditions such as ADD or Autism. After noticing the significant changes to her daughter's health without dairy, she started to encourage the parents of her clients to take their kids off of it. When I would talk with her she would say, "I feel my clients would focus better if they would go off dairy".

I do not want to put down the dairy industry! I am from Wisconsin! But I do think we need to look at the issue of what foods we really can or can't eat. Cow dairy is one we need to be careful of, especially with our children. The issue may not be with the cow milk insomuch as it is in how the cows are raised. Whatever chemicals or hormones are given to the cows gets into the milk and then we consume that. Some of my patients do fine with organic dairy products, but if they get the non-organic they experience adverse symptoms.

If my friend is starting to see extensive correlations between foods like cow dairy and behavior in children, and believes strongly that it is a serious problem, consider taking your child off it and see what happens!

Here is what I have taught patients to do if their Child Starts To Get Sick:

1. Remove offending food allergens. Your child may have gotten exposed to a food their body doesn't like. Even temporary removal of foods hard on digestion can get your child better faster. The most common foods that I see causing problems in children are dairy, eggs, wheat (gluten), and sugar.

2. Keep sugar (processed and most fruits) out of their diet. Antioxidant-rich fruits like berries are fine; they are lower in sugars and higher in Vitamin C.

3. Integrative Therapeutics V-clear is a great anti-viral homeopathic; even a few drops throughout the day is perfect. This product will not interfere with any medications.

4. Rest.

⤜ 12 ⤏
Fever

Fever is defined as an oral temperature greater than 100.4 F (38 C). Fever starts when the regulating system (located in the hypothalamus) is reset to a higher temperature via the action of the signaling molecules in the immune system (Chapter 6). In other words, something tells the white blood cells that there is a virus, bacteria, or other offending agent in the body, and the cells respond by telling other cells something is wrong (the ping-pong/Internet signaling process from Chapter 6). This signal goes to the brain (the hypothalamus) and triggers a regulating center to change the body temperature.

The following is a list of conditions that tend to be associated with a Low-grade Fever (fever 100 or less):

Autoimmune Diseases

Cancer

Ear Infections

Infections (i.e. Cold or Flu)

Food Sensitivity Reactions

Reactions to Medications

The following is a list of conditions that tend to be associated with a High-grade Fever (fever 102 or higher):

Bronchitis

Infections

Pneumonia

Fever must be judged carefully. Fever of 104 and greater can be dangerous: if that happens, go to the ER immediately. On one of my trips to Nepal to volunteer medical care, I saw a six-year old who was mentally and physically handicapped. He required 24-hour care. In taking his case I learned that he was not born with any handicaps: he had been born totally normal. He had a very high fever two years prior that had left him incapacitated. His mother had not been able to get him to medical care.

Fever is Diagnosed via:

Temperature Above Your Baseline Normal

✚ Conventional Medical Treatment Options for High and Low-grade Fever include:

Medications that Lower Fever (i.e. Tylenol)

Antibiotics

Electrolyte IVs

Fluids

Rest

* **Alternative Medical Treatment Options include:**

Herbs

Electrolyte Drinks/Mixes

Fluids

Rest

❂ Naturopathic Medicine, Treating the Cause:

Naturopathic standards are similar to Conventional treatment options if the fever is 104 or above. If above 104, your Naturopathic Doctor will refer you to the ER, just as a Conventional Doctor will. If the fever is less than 104, the Naturopath will be supporting your immune system while Treating the Cause.

If fever is not from a cold or flu, it takes detective work on behalf of the Naturopath to identify what the cause is. This process is extremely important and takes teamwork. You need to disclose as much information as you can to your physician so they may better be able to identify the cause(s). Once this is done, the cause is treated (not the fever). Treating the Cause will shift the fever, bringing your body temperature back to normal range.

Most people will treat themselves or their children with fever-reducing Tylenol. I don't recommend it only because fever is a good thing when it is not too high (not close to or above 104). Fever stimulates the signaling process within the immune system so that your body can better respond to the virus or bacteria: heat activates white blood cells and signaling molecules (Chapter 6).

Treating the Cause with the Power of Belief:

Any deviation in your temperature from your normal is a signal that something is not right with your immune system. I have a patient who has become very good at listening to her body, and she knows immediately when she needs to call me. She had an experience once where her body temperature dropped suddenly. After I assessed her symptoms, I sent her to the ER for an immediate evaluation. As she pulled into the ER, her temperature suddenly spiked.

She was diagnosed with a TIA, which is a small block of a blood vessel in her brain: her body told her things were off by the drop in temperature (she had no other symptoms). This patient is totally healthy and fine because we caught a problem early and she received the treatment she needed. If she didn't believe in listening to her body, we may have missed this.

**Here is what I have taught my patients to do
if they start to feel a change in Body Temperature:**

1. Call me so we can discuss symptoms.

2. Use Ferrum phosphoricum homeopathic for high fevers related to cold/flu. Integrative Therapeutics V-clear may also help, especially if the fever is caused by a virus.

3. Use a sitz bath at a cool temperature with Epsom salts.

4. Think through what may have caused a fever to start: has anything changed in diet/lifestyle?

❧ 13 ❧
Airway Diseases

Airway diseases include lung cancer, emphysema, chronic obstructive pulmonary disease (COPD), asthma, bronchitis, or pneumonia. These conditions have similar symptoms such as cough or shortness of breath.

Airway Diseases are Diagnosed via:

Lung Function Testing by a Pulmonologist

Low Density CT to Screen for Cancer

Blood Work

Symptom Presentation at Physical Exam

Sputum Culture

X-ray

Even though similar tools are used for diagnostic purposes, treatment varies with disease.

✚ Conventional Medical Treatment Options include:

Oxygen

Medications (i.e. Antibiotics, Steroids, Inhalers)

Rest

Physical Therapy

Removal of Tumor or Chemotherapy/Radiation

❊ Alternative Medical Treatment Options include:

Acupuncture/Massage

Herbs

Vitamins/Minerals

✪ Naturopathic Medicine, Treating the Cause:

The lungs are sensitive to anything that causes inflammation. Environmental toxins are a major source of inflammation and this tends to be what most physicians think of when they start to treat lung diseases: air pollutants are the most common source of toxins to the lungs, and this can include cigarette smoke, automobile exhaust, or cleaning product fumes.

From work with my patients I have learned other causes of lung inflammation such as:

Adrenal Fatigue (Chapter 8)

Chemotherapy/Radiation

Food Sensitivities

Low Glutathione (Chapter 4)

Low Magnesium Levels

I approach lung disease cases by taking a very careful history because the causes listed above can have similar symptoms (such as shortness of breath). I have to tease out where the problem is, when it started, or what it started from. After I have a clear understanding of that, I will start a treatment protocol with my patient.

Here is a case as an example:

Patient came to my office for shortness of breath. She had experienced this for several years. Complicating her picture was high blood pressure, depression, anxiety, and insomnia. She was not able to sleep without medication use and she would cry easily. She was on four different anti-psychotic medications when I met her. She needed Ambien to help her sleep and HCTZ for the high blood pressure. She was not able to function without constant oxygen support via a nose feed: she carried her oxygen tank with her.

After taking a careful history and seeing her a few times, I decided the root cause was most likely adrenal dysfunction due to long-standing stressors that had started months PRIOR. I started her on my Adrenal herbs and weekly acupuncture. We began to see changes by about week five. She first noticed that she would wake at night without her oxygen on (she took it off while sleeping which she had never done before). Her oxygen and blood pressure levels began to stabilize, she had less weepiness, and was sleeping better.

This patient had underlying adrenal hormone dysfunction that caused her symptoms (Chapter 8).

Treating the Cause with the Power of Belief:

I have a pediatric brother and sister who struggle with chronic coughs and cold/flu. I started working with these patients over a year ago, at a time when they were coughing almost constantly, and would not improve from Conventional treatments such as inhalers. I started with identification of any possible sources of inflammation that would affect the lungs such as allergens in their environment, food sensitivities, and genetic weaknesses (such as low glutathione from Chapter 4).

The parents took gluten out of their kids' diets and saw significant lessoning in frequency of the cough. We worked on supporting their immune systems and liver detoxification pathways (the lungs are high in glutathione) and noticed the kids did not get as sick as often.

The oldest of the two children still had a cough when he exercised, so I decided to refer him to see Dr. Mike Knapp, NMD, who is very good at picking the right homeopathic remedy. Homeopathy can help shift stubborn symptoms.

Dr. Knapp did pick the right remedy at the conclusion of the initial consultation, but it stimulated a bit of a healing crisis in the cough (meaning, the symptoms got worse at initial dosing of the remedy). The parents stayed the course even though it seemed like the child was worse; in a short period of time the cough decreased significantly and his breathing was better than it had been.

If these parents did not trust and believe, and activate the power of their believing, they would have quit the homeopathic remedy too soon, and we would not have seen such a rapid resolution of symptoms.

Here is what I have taught my patients to do if they struggle with an Airway Disease:

1. Be patient and continue to work to identify what may be aggravating the lung tissues.

2. Eliminate foods like wheat and dairy from the diet. Cow dairy is notorious for creating inflammation in the lungs and sinuses.

3. Keep processed sugar low to non-existent in the diet. Sugar promotes inflammation (Chapter 15).

4. Use acupuncture to tone lung chi.

5. Keep the adrenals healthy. The adrenal glands regulate the energy of the lungs (clinical observation).

6. Use IV or my sublingual glutathione if levels are low (Chapter 4).

7. Keep magnesium levels high via a diet high in greens (green foods have good levels of magnesium). If that is not enough, I like the magnesium by Thorne (cal/mag citrate powder). Or, an IV will help get magnesium into tissues when immediate increases are needed. Magnesium is a bronchodilator (it allows bronchioles to relax, which helps decrease lung tissue spasms).

❧ 14 ❧
Urinary Tract Infections

In the U.S. every year, 1,200 women and 30 men per 100,000 experience urinary tract infections (UTI), which is inflammation of the bladder due to bacterial overgrowth. Symptoms include urinary frequency, blood in the urine, incontinence, low back pain, pelvic pain, or fever.

Urinary tract infections (UTI) are Diagnosed via:
Urinalysis
Urine culture
Cystourethrogram
Pyelogram
CT of Abdomen/Pelvis
Ultrasound

A culture will diagnose a UTI, but if the symptoms become chronic, other imaging studies or blood work will be ordered (www.mdconsult.com/das/search/results/403746318-13?searchId=1411701951&kw=UTI&area=FirstConsult&set=1&bbSearchType=single).

✚ Conventional Medical Treatment Options include:
Antibiotics
Bladder Scope (to Rule Out Cancer)
Increased Water Intake

✳ Alternative Medical Treatment Options include:
Cranberry Juice
Increased Water Intake
Herbs

✪ Naturopathic Medicine, Treating the Cause:
Urinary tract infections manifest as a result of an unbalanced system that then allows bacteria to overgrow.

Causes of the Imbalance include:

Acidic Diet	Chronic Stress	Processed Sugar Intake
Hormone Changes	Spermicides or Condoms	

I recommend my patients keep their body slightly alkaline. This is most easily accomplished by consumption of veggies and berries while avoiding (as much as possible) processed sugars, grains, or alcohol (alcoholic beverages are very sugary). Processed foods, alcohol, and excessive protein intake create what is called an acidic pH in your body fluids. Veggies, fruits (berries preferably), and a balance of protein in the diet (protein intake at 20% or less) creates an "alkaline" environment (a pH that is just right for your body). Just the right pH keeps bacterial growth at a minimum.

Low vaginal estrogen can trigger a UTI. High systemic (body-wide) estrogen can do the same. I always check estrogen levels via blood work in patients struggling with chronic UTIs. If estrogen is high relative to the other hormones (high relative to testosterone and progesterone), I prescribe Indoplex by Integrative Therapeutics, 1-2 daily. This is a great supplement supporting estrogen metabolism and is derived from broccoli. If vaginal estrogen is low (common in postmenopausal women) I may prescribe a vaginal estrogen cream. Getting estrogen levels in balance is key in the prevention of urinary tract infections.

Stress elevates cortisol (Chapter 8). Cortisol suppresses the immune system when it has been elevated too long. When this happens, bacteria can overgrow and the consumption of processed sugars will worsen it. If a patient is dealing with a lot of stress I generally recommend avoiding sugars especially during these times (I recommend avoidance of sugar all the time but especially during stress).

Cranberry juice may or may not resolve a UTI. Unfortunately, cranberry routinely shows as a sensitivity on food tests. For these patients, consuming cranberry actually creates inflammation, which can exacerbate a UTI. For those with sensitivities to cranberry, I recommend the supplement D-mannose, the constituent in cranberry useful against E. coli (Tambouri 2005) but without all the other cranberry ingredients that may contribute to inflammation.

It is best to get a urine culture done first to see what strain of bacteria may be contributing to the UTI. Patients can find themselves in the hospital if an early UTI is not treated properly (as the infection may jump to the kidneys), so I always use my clinical judgment to decide whether or not a treatment such as an herb is appropriate. Sometimes a combination of herbs and antibiotics is best.

Treating the Cause with the Power of Belief:

One of my patients has dealt with chronic urinary tract infections for years. She had been on and off antibiotics for almost a decade, and by the time she came to see me felt like she was "overwhelmed" with medicines and not getting any better. We took a look at her overall lifestyle as I discussed above (diet, alcohol consumption, protein intake) and she made some changes. She started with lessoning alcohol consumption.

Shortly after we began to make changes, she started to get another UTI. Her conviction in the healing power of her body was so strong that for the first time she decided to avoid antibiotics, quit alcohol (rather than slowly taper it), and ride out the UTI. She decided to use herbs to support her body's ability to lower the bacterial activity; I blended some herbs for her and within a few days her UTI was totally gone. This was a huge shift for her, as normally they lasted for 2-3 weeks. She believed in the healing power of her body and in the power of herbal medicines!

This is what I have taught my patients to do if they start to get a UTI:

1. Start on their herbal medicine UTI blend right away.

2. Eliminate sources of sugar. Viruses and bacteria become increasingly active if you eat processed sugars (clinical experience).

3. Drink liver supportive herbs such as dandelion root tea. The liver has to process all inflammation out of the body. It will need extra support during any kind of acute inflammatory process.

4. Get an acupuncture treatment to facilitate the movement of energy.

5. Use antibiotics if necessary, as a UTI can get to the kidneys if it spreads.

ༀ 15 ༀ
Insulin Resistance, Diabetes & Metabolic Syndrome

Insulin resistance is impaired metabolism of glucose (www.mdconsult.com/daspd-md/body/403903122-13/1412417039?type=med&eid=9-u1.0-_1_mt_5080901), while Type II Diabetes is the loss of pancreatic cell function (which normally regulates insulin production). When insulin resistance has a mix of impaired glucose metabolism with pancreatic cell function loss, it may be called "metabolic syndrome".

Metabolic Syndrome and Insulin Resistance are Diagnosed via:
Blood Work including Lipids and Insulin
Blood Pressure Screenings
Waist-to-hip Ratios to Evaluate and Diagnose Obesity
Fasting Glucose

Both of these conditions are associated with diseases including:
Cardiovascular Disease
Coronary Artery Disease
Type II Diabetes

✚ Conventional Medical Treatment Options include:
Medications (i.e. Insulin, Metformin)
Exercise
Diet Changes (Reduce Fat/Carb Intake)
Aspirin

✳ Alternative Medical Treatment Options include:
Diet Changes
Exercise
Supplements for Blood Sugar (i.e. Chromium, Bitter Melon)

❂ Naturopathic Medicine, Treating the Cause:
Blood sugar diseases can result from almost any imbalance in any part of your body's normal biochemical functions (Chapters 1-9). However, in my research I am finding that sugar issues stem from inflammatory processes stimulated via your immune system (Johnson and Olefsky 2013). And if unchecked, the inflammation that caused the insulin resistance can lead to the development of Type II Diabetes.

According to Johnson, Olefsky, and my clinical experience,
insulin resistance leads to diabetes via three mechanisms:
Inflammation
Dysbiosis (Changes to Gut Bacteria)
Low Omega Oil Levels (Chapter 1)

Here is how inflammation, gut bacterial changes and fats can cause insulin resistance:

Step One: Fat and sugar levels increase WITHIN the cell. Omega oil levels drop and hydrogenated or trans fat levels increase (Chapter 1).

Step Two: Gut bacteria levels change. Good bacteria such as acidophilus decrease, possibly from lack of dietary intake. Stress can change gut bacterial levels because of changes in adrenal cortisol levels (clinical experience).

Step Three: Macrophages (Chapter 6) in the immune system notice the increase in bad fat/sugars and the decrease in good gut bacteria.

Step Four: Macrophages start to signal to other macrophages via signaling molecules that something is off in the body's balance (the ping-pong ball/Internet signal analogy from Chapter 6).

Step Five: Macrophages build up INSIDE the cells in response to the high bad fat/sugar and changing bacterial levels.

Step Six: Macrophages keep signaling that the balance is off, triggering an inflammatory cascade.

Step Seven: Chronic inflammation leads to diseases such as insulin resistance or diabetes.

Summary: The immune system macrophages respond in the same way to sugars as they do bad fats. Macrophages build up INSIDE cells and then start signaling inflammation.

Sugars can also be stuck to the surface of cells, called "HgA1c". This HgA1c (hemoglobin A1c) is measured to evaluate and diagnose diabetes and insulin resistance, but I am checking it in a majority of my patients even if their fasting blood sugar levels are normal. I am theorizing that HgA1c promotes inflammation in the same way that the build up of macrophages inside the cell does.

I recommend that my patients scrutinize their diets to look for any hidden processed sugars. Most people are surprised with the amount of sugars they are actually consuming. Smoothie fasting is a great way to get the immune system to shift once the processed sugars are at a minimum. I recommend patients throw in a blender some greens, berries (organic), and some healthy fat oils (such as coconut oil, 1 tbsp is fine) and pull the protein out of their diet for one to five days, then go back to normal eating habits. The drop in protein levels and addition of high-dose antioxidants seems to create a very positive shift in the immune system that starts to lower inflammation. I have seen patients' sugar levels decrease with this kind of diet, especially if the patient does smoothie fasting regularly, perhaps a few times a month for anywhere from one to five days. For some, one day a week is enough to make them feel great, get blood sugars in balance, lose weight, and drop inflammation.

Treating the Cause with the Power of Belief:

I have a patient in her 60s who was very concerned about her weight, blood pressure, cholesterol, and blood sugar levels. She had weight around her middle and she tended to hover around 170 pounds; she felt that was at least 40 pounds too much for her body frame. She "tried everything" to lose weight and manage all her health conditions but without medications she was not able to improve anything.

When I evaluated her case, I found that all of her conditions stemmed from chronic gut inflammation. She was very sensitive to foods and stress. She would eat the smallest amount of a food that she was sensitive to and she would put on at least 6 pounds and have accompanying abdominal pain, bloating, or gas. As I put her case together, I began to realize she was most likely experiencing overactive macrophages. The macrophages were signaling to other immune cells that there was overriding inflammation (or foods that triggered inflammation); and that message continued to other macrophages, causing her symptoms.

She was worried my diagnosis was wrong because it seemed a bit far-fetched to her, but she decided to believe and trust. We tested all her food sensitivities via blood and she committed to avoiding them as best she could. She pulled processed sugars out of her diet and she started working with a personal trainer on an exercise regime. The weight stayed the same for several months and she would email me that she felt this would not work but asked what I thought? I was convinced that with more time the immune system would start to shift and I was right. She stuck with the exercise program, she stuck with her diet, and she set her mind that she could do this.

She did!

Within a few weeks more she began to lose weight. At the time I wrote this she had dropped her weight 30 pounds!

Here is what I have taught my patients to do
if they have Blood Sugar Metabolism Problems:

1. Get processed sugars and non-Omega oils out of the diet. Oils that have been fried and packaged seem to create a lot of health problems for patients (clinical experience); this includes chips and nuts that have been fried, roasted, or baked.

2. Start and stick to an exercise program; build the program into your lifestyle and do something you enjoy.

3. Support the liver's ability to process inflammation. Castor oil packs are great at doing this (Chapter 35).

4. Increase antioxidant-rich foods in the diet (these are the colorful fruits and veggies such as berries or greens; these foods lower inflammation).

5. Fast from protein. Protein promotes inflammation via signaling molecules (Chapter 6).

∞ 16 ∞
Obesity

Sixty-six percent of U.S. adults are overweight (www.mdconsult.com/das/pdxmd/body/421094632-3/0?type=med&eid=9-u1.0-_1_mt_1016556). Obesity is defined as body mass that exceeds weight-to-height ratio (www.en.wikipedia.org/wiki/Obesity).

Obesity is Diagnosed via:
Body Mass Index (Calculated as a Function of Weight/Height)
Waist-to-hip Ratio and Circumference

It is often associated with conditions including:

Arthritis	High Blood Pressure
Cardiovascular Disease	Sleep Apnea
Genetics	Medication Sensitivity
Gout	Thyroid Disorders

✚ Conventional Medical Treatment Options include:
Counseling
Diet Changes
Exercise
Surgery
Medications (i.e. Anti-depressants)

✳ Alternative Medical Treatment Options include:
Diet Changes
Exercise
Blood-sugar Regulating Supplements
Appetite Suppressant Supplements
Metabolism "Boosters" as Supplements

✪ Naturopathic Medicine, Treating the Cause:
In my opinion, obesity results from factors such as low Omega levels (Chapter 1), too much stress (Chapter 8), too much protein (Chapter 6), and too many processed sugars in the diet (Chapter 15). All of these encourage the body to put on inflammatory weight, especially if there is not enough exercise or balancing of the adrenal glands (Chapter 8).

Some patients lose weight by behavior modifications (i.e. increasing exercise or changing diet) while some do not. If you are one of those who does not see a benefit with exercise and diet changes, I suggest you read Chapter 15 on insulin resistance (pay attention to the discussion on the immune system). It is also important to remove food sensitivities and sugary foods because they create inflammation. Inflammation keeps weight on (clinical observation).

I recommend:

- Exercise.
- Diet Changes (Remove Food Sensitivities/Sugar).
- Treat Underlying Inflammatory Condition.
- Address Hormonal Conditions (i.e. Hypothyroidism/Adrenal Dysfunction/Elevated Estrogen).
- Increase Antioxidants in the Diet (I have noticed that berries are really good at helping balance blood sugar).

Treating the Cause with the Power of Belief:

I had a patient with extensive osteoarthritic joint pain and obesity. Initially she had gained weight when she was unable to exercise anymore (due to the pain). Over the course of a few years she put on 50 pounds. She came to me at a time in her life when she felt she was "at wits end about my weight" and needed to walk with a walker to help her move.

After a careful history taking, I asked her to start by the elimination of dairy and wheat from her diet. I see that both foods, whether they show up on food sensitivity testing or not, cause a lot of pain/inflammation. I think they cause problems because they are genetically modified. I also checked her hormones and her testosterone was actually very low. I added a small topical dose as a cream and had her apply it daily.

I hardly recognized her when she came back in a few months later! No walker! She had lost 20 pounds (thus far) and this increased her mobility as well as decreased pain.

Here is what I have taught my patients to do if they start to Put On Weight or struggle to Lose Weight:

1. Identify any possible sources of inflammation.

2. Check hormone levels; high estrogen can keep on weight.

3. Keep thyroid levels balanced.

4. Exercise regularly. Find something enjoyable to do.

5. Avoid processed sugar.

6. Eat a diet high in antioxidants.

7. Keep toxic emotions out of the body/spirit. Difficult emotional times can put on weight as they change the adrenal output of cortisol (Chapters 8 and 9).

8. Protein fast (Chapter 6).

❧ 17 ❧
Heart Disease

Heart Disease is a blanket term for diseases such as:

Angina	Mitral/Tricuspid Regurgitation
Arrhythmias	Prolapsed Heart Valves
Coronary (Heart) Vessel Blocks	Pulmonary Hypertension
High Blood Pressure	Rheumatic Fever
Hyperlipidemia	Septal Defects
Affecting Heart Valves/Vessels	Stroke
Illness	Tachycardia
Ischemia	

Heart disease is a leading cause of death in the United States, UK, Canada, and Australia. Symptoms include palpitations, shortness of breath, skin tone changes, fatigue, or wheezing. However, some patients may not have any symptoms (www.md-consult.com/das/pdxmd/body/402582560-4/1407380125?type=med&eid=9-u1.0-_1_mt_1014218).

Heart Disease is Diagnosed via:

Stress test

EKG

Echocardiogram

CBC/CMP in Blood Work

Kidney Function Tests

✛ Conventional Medical Treatment Options include:

Medications, Beta Blockers (i.e. Metoprolol)

Medications, ACE Inhibitors (i.e. Lisinopril)

Medications, Diuretics (i.e. HCTZ)

Ablation

Heart Replacement

Pacemakers

Anticoagulant Medications (i.e. Warfarin, Aspirin)

Valve Replacement

Physical Therapy

Medications (i.e. Statin Drugs like Simvastatin)

Oxygen

Medications, Vasodilators (i.e. Nitroglycerin)

Coronary Bypass

Revascularization

✳ **Alternative Medical Treatment Options include:**

Herbs (i.e. Hawthorne)

Acupuncture

Supplements (i.e. CoQ10, Red Yeast Rice, L-carnitine)

Diet Changes

Exercise

⊙ **Naturopathic Medicine, Treating the Cause:**

Heart disease often starts from an imbalance of fats in the diet (Chapter 1), as well as miscommunication of neurotransmitters (Chapter 7), dysfunction of the mitochondria (Chapter 3), inflammation (Chapter 6), and an inability or unwillingness to listen to the heart's desires (Chapter 9).

The heart is a large muscle. It requires calcium to contract, magnesium to relax, CoQ10 for energy production (Chapters 2 and 3), and the nervous system to regulate heartbeat (Chapter 7). If something causes calcium, magnesium, or CoQ10 levels to drop, any type of heart disease may manifest depending on your genetics. Altered nervous system function, inflammation (Chapter 6), low antioxidant load (Chapter 5), or increased LDL cholesterol may be some factors that alter these nutrients.

Nutrients taken to support heart function need to be taken in balanced doses. For example, daily supplemental calcium levels should not exceed 1000 to 1200 mg daily or it will actually contribute to heart disease (Steriti 2010). Too often I see Conventional Doctors putting patients on MORE calcium if they don't see results on a standard dose. Don't do that. More is not always better. Too much calcium "interferes with magnesium absorption, increases the potential for clot formation with vasospasm, and increases oxidative stress" (Steriti 2010).

Here is a patient case to illustrate my point. This case also demonstrates the complexity in treating the heart.

A 70 year-old retired diesel truck driver had been on high blood pressure medications for several years. In taking his history, I learned he never had any problems with his heart until 2006. In 2006, he experienced a sudden onset of pain that radiated to his left arm; he went to his physician who found blockages in several arteries on the left side of his heart. He was treated with two stents and a pacemaker. After the surgery, he developed shortness of breath and chest tightness worse with exertion. His ejection fraction with the pacemaker remained below normal at 35-40%

In June 2012:

• I prescribed castor oil/magnesium oil packs over the heart. (I learned this trick from Dr. Weiss, a Naturopath/Cardiologist in Scottsdale, AZ). I had the patient rub both oils on the skin over the heart, cover with a thin cloth, then cover with a hot water bottle and rest for 10-15 minutes. The oils decrease inflammation and increase effectiveness of the heart's ability to pump blood.

• I ordered specialty lab Genova Diagnostics blood testing to evaluate mitochondria function and levels of inflammatory markers. His mitochondrial function was overactive and he was positive for IL-1B (one of the signalers, see Chapter 6).

• I recommended infrared sauna at home a few days a week for 20 minutes a session.

• I recommended Thorne Heavy Metal Support and Solvent Remover.

• I recommended increased antioxidants in diet.

• I prescribed sublingual L-carnitine/L-taurine/B12 sublingual lozenges compounded by Civic Center Pharmacy in Scottsdale, AZ.

At the August 2012-September 2012 follow-ups:

His shortness of breath was gone, but he was still having some chest discomforts and was complaining of fatigue. He had started the sauna and was noticing a "stinky" smell coming off his skin after the sauna.

• I prescribed IV magnesium.

• I prescribed liver support (with my Immune Formula which contains a great deal of both liver supportive and anti-inflammatory herbs).

At the October 2012 follow-up:

His blood pressure was coming down from the 180s to the 160-130s (systolic, top number). He was still experiencing some chest pressure.

• I added sublingual lozenge of magnesium/CoQ10 (compounded by Civic Center Pharmacy).

- I added ginger (helps lower inflammation and promotes circulation).

At the November 2012 follow-up:

He shared that his chest discomfort was nearly gone. His blood pressure was staying around 160-130s (systolic). He noticed that the blood pressure dropped the most with the castor oil/magnesium packs over his heart.

- At this point I recommended that he reschedule with his cardiologist so we could evaluate his ejection fraction. His levels did indeed improve! Results are in the next Figure 19.

Figure 19

Left Ventricle: Systolic function is abnormal. Ejection fraction is 55-60%. Moderate concentric hypertrophy is present. Apex is akinetic.

Figure 19. Cardiologist results showing improved ejection fraction results.

Treating the Cause with the Power of Belief:

Most patients know when something is wrong with their heart. The heart has relatively unmistakable beats when the electrical conduction has changed.

The heart is in delicate balance with the rest of the body. I had a patient who was doing well on our Naturopathic Plan but I met him too late in his life. He had worked with me closely for several months until we figured out the causes of his heart disease; after that point I rarely heard from him as he was improving by leaps and bounds as he applied Naturopathic Principles to his lifestyle. Months later he called to tell me he felt really tired, which was a new symptom. He was not sure what it was from, as his heart rate and blood pressure were holding steady at normal levels.

I told him to come to see me right away, but he never made it to his appointment. I called him to see if he was on his way, but he did not answer. I began to feel concerned but assumed something must have come up that delayed his drive (he lived an hour away).

I got a call a few hours later from his wife to let me know he passed away on his way in to see me. What a devastating call that was. The good thing is that I had taught him to listen to his body and to know when to call. He knew something was not right; his heart ended up giving out on him during his drive to see me.

As I write this I still feel devastated, as I had much appreciation for this patient: he always used to tell me my research and work "is quite a kick, Doc". I wish he was still here, but I am pleased he did reach out even though he had not been having any direct heart symptoms: he believed his body would tell him when something was not right, and he followed through to take the best care of himself that he could. He will be missed.

Here is what I have taught my patients to do if they have Heart Disease:

1. Find a good cardiologist to work with. More often than not heart disease patients can benefit from proper management of medications if they are needed. Once biochemical processes outlined in Part One have been altered or become stressed and the heart suffers, it can be difficult to reverse. Therefore, medications may be necessary to extend life.

2. Work slowly into an exercise program or work with a personal trainer.

3. Keep magnesium and CoQ10 levels up.

4. Only use herbs if prescribed by your Naturopathic Doctor. I don't advocate the use of herbs unless they are prescribed by someone knowledgeable about them, as many of the herbals will interact negatively with the prescription medications. My patients know to ask me before they think to add an herb. Hawthorne, for example, is good for the heart but it increases the heart's ability to pump out blood: if you are on a heart-rate monitoring medication that may not be the best choice. Hawthorne may also affect the way your body metabolizes medications.

❦ 18 ❦
High Blood Pressure (HTN)

High blood pressure affects 65 million adults in the U.S. annually. It is defined as elevated blood pressure in two or more visits to your physician. Systolic blood pressure (the top number) will be above 140 and diastolic (the bottom number) above 80. Patients may be asymptomatic (without symptoms) when blood pressure is high or may suffer from headaches, ringing in the ears, vision disturbances, gait disturbances, or water weight fluctuations (www.mdconsult.com/das/search/results/403746318-9?searchId=1411691985&kw=HTN&area=FirstConsult&set=1&bbSearchType=single).

High Blood Pressure is Diagnosed via:
Two or More Elevated Blood Pressure Readings

Kidney Function Tests

Kidney Ultrasound/CT Scan of Abdomen

EKG

Stress Test

Thyroid Blood Work

Cancer Screening

CT Angiogram

Chest X-ray

High blood pressure can be associated with many other conditions. Therefore, it is important to get a full workup from your primary care doctor; if deeper pathology is suspected, you will be referred to a specialist such as a heart or kidney doctor. Both the heart and the kidneys help regulate blood pressure.

Conditions that tend to be associated with High Blood Pressure include:
Thyroid Disorders

Kidney Diseases

Tumors

Adrenal Diseases

Constriction of the Aorta

Atherosclerosis

✚ Conventional Medical Treatment Options include:
Medications (i.e. "Water Pills", such as HCTZ)

Medications that Alter Heart Rate (i.e. ACE Inhibitors, Calcium Channel Blockers)

Managing diseases associated with the high blood pressure

Eliminating Alcohol

Exercise

Smoking Cessation

✳ Alternative Medical Treatment Options include:

Herbs

Supplements to Affect Heart Rate/Relaxation

❂ Naturopathic Medicine, Treating the Cause:

High blood pressure can come about from any change to the biochemical process discussed in Part One (Chapters 1-9). That being said, many patients who have high blood pressure have low magnesium levels. Your heart uses calcium to contract (pump blood) and magnesium to relax (allowing it to fill with blood). People today tend to eat very few foods that have magnesium in them (green foods have high levels of magnesium).

I tell patients to get a liquid or powder magnesium supplement. Stress depletes magnesium levels very quickly (because magnesium is used to create neurotransmitters and hormones, Chapters 7 and 8). Today a patient with high blood pressure told me her MD put her on magnesium but it didn't work. I told her it didn't most likely because she was on the wrong form (she was on tablets). In my opinion, tablet supplements rarely absorb, as I don't usually see them create positive changes.

With hypertension, it is very important to rule out any other disease or condition. For example, high blood pressure can result from kidney or liver diseases, abdominal pain, chronic migraines, high cortisol levels (Chapter 8), cancer, medication side effects, or supplement side effects.

To Treat the Cause:

- Use liquid or powdered magnesium (I like the calcium/magnesium citrate by Thorne).
- Increase intake of mineral-rich veggies (greens especially).
- See your Naturopathic Physician for vitamin IV therapies high in magnesium.
- Practice stress reduction.
- Lower toxin exposure (mercury competes with magnesium within the cell, Crinnion 2004-5).
- Pull trans fats and hydrogenated oils out of your diet (Chapter 1).

Treating the Cause with the Power of Belief:

I have a patient who was adamantly opposed to being on the medication Lisinopril for her high blood pressure. She came to me hoping we could find a way to get her off it.

At the first visit I suggested she try the formulation by Mountain Peaks called Heart Tension (created by one of my colleagues). I never use this formula in isolation as I still work with patients to identify the cause(s) of their high blood pressure. I started her on this while we worked together to treat her as a whole person—her adrenals, mind/body connection, and diet. As we did treatments such as acupuncture, diet changes, and increased mineral levels, she tapered slowly off the Lisinopril. Within a few months, she was totally off the Lisinopril and found that she only needed one capsule of the herbs a day to keep her blood pressure at a perfect level!

Here is what I have taught my patients to do if they have High Blood Pressure:

1. High blood pressure always has a cause and it is important to find it. The heart is in delicate balance with the rest of the body. I am not against medications (drugs), but I am against bad prescribing of said medications: oftentimes patients are put on too many medications or a blend of them that is actually hard on the heart, kidneys, or liver.

2. High blood pressure is oftentimes a reflection of low magnesium levels. Magnesium allows muscles to relax (while calcium contributes to contraction); most of us are lower on magnesium than calcium.

3. Take 20 mg daily (oral) of CoQ10. CoQ10 is fat-soluble and should be taken with food.

4. If you get ringing in your ears, feel flushed, dizzy, or have any other sudden onset of symptoms, call right away or go to the ER. Blood pressure, if it elevates too high too fast, can be considered an emergency or be a signal that something else is wrong.

❧ 19 ❧
High Cholesterol Levels

Fifty percent of the U.S. adult population has high cholesterol levels. Men more than women tend to have high cholesterol. An elevation in cholesterol may lead to increased risk of arterial diseases such as atherosclerosis www.mdconsult.com/das/pdxmd/body/421209396-4/1467106703?type=med&eid=9-u1.0-_1_mt_1014732). Although cholesterol is blamed for atherosclerosis, it is actually a very useful molecule. For example, it is used to make hormones such as estrogen or testosterone. It also transports fats to cells for energy and cell membrane construction (Chapter 1).

Cholesterol is made up of various types, primarily HDL and LDL. HDL is considered "good cholesterol" because it circulates in the bloodstream and collects fatty cholesterol molecules. As it collects these molecules, it brings them to the cells to see if the cells need them. LDLs are leftover particles from the action of HDL: the fats/cholesterol in HDL get used up and broken into leftovers the cells don't need at the time. The leftovers are termed "remnants". The remnants are the LDLs. LDLs have various types, called "remnant" or "low density" (Guyton and Hall 2000). These LDLs contribute to cardiovascular diseases.

High Cholesterol is Diagnosed via:
Blood Work

✚ Conventional Medical Treatment Options include:
Cholesterol-lowering Medications (i.e. Statin Drugs, Thyroid Medications)
Dietary Modifications
Exercise

✳ Alternative Medical Treatment Options include:
Herbs
Dietary Modifications
Exercise
Supplements (i.e. Red Yeast Rice or Niacinamide)

◎ Naturopathic Medicine, Treating the Cause:
High cholesterol is partly due to low levels of Omega fats in the diet (Chapter 1), low exercise levels, low antioxidant levels, high sugars in the diet, and age (clinical experience).

I have seen a lot of patients who experience an increase in their cholesterol levels as they age. Current medical standards of care dictate patients go on cholesterol-lowering medications if their total cholesterol is greater than 200. Cholesterol is used to make steroid hormones—the hormones DHEA, cortisol, estrogen, progesterone, and testosterone. The adrenals are responsible for making these hormones (Chapter 8). If you lower your cholesterol too much there may not be enough left to make hormones (my theory).

For my patients, I check to see what types of cholesterol they have because the total cholesterol number is not very useful in and of itself: I order a specialty lab test by SpectraCell called the Lipoprotein Particle test. This test gives a breakdown of the types of cholesterol particles, including the ones called remnant and low density (Figure 20).

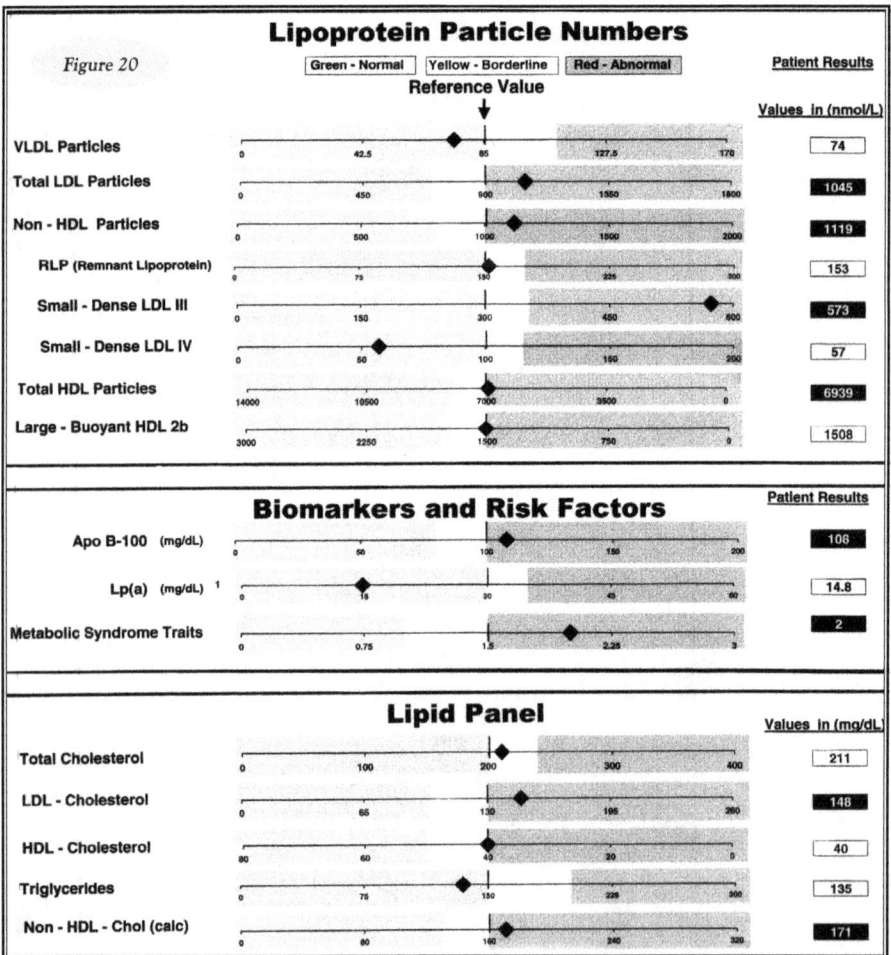

Figure 20. Lipoprotein test. Pay particular attention to the diamonds.

Your blood vessels are very sensitive to environmental toxins, especially cigarette smoke: the inner layer of blood vessels will get micro-tears from cigarette smoke or other toxins (Crinnion 2004-5). When this happens, the remnant and low-density LDL particles start to get trapped in the area of the micro-tears, leading to a build-up of cholesterol in the walls of blood vessels. After this point, immune cells respond to the presence of the fats and a cascade of inflammation starts (Chapter 6). This is more of the problem of atherosclerosis than just elevated cholesterol itself.

If a Lipoprotein test result shows a high number of remnant or low-density LDL particles, I will recommend the patient go on a no sugar, high antioxidant, anti-inflammatory diet. I will also prescribe supplementation of fish oils or niacin (wax matrix niacin is the best form to lower low-density LDLs, Swanson 2013). I am also finding that my Pitcher Plant Tincture is absolutely amazing at helping regulate inflammatory reactions (patient symptoms such as body aches decrease with this formulation, see my website for details). I am suspecting the pitcher plant has an impact on the ping-pong ball/Internet signaling from the immune system that creates inflammation (Chapter 6).

If you only look at total cholesterol and not at the individual particles, you may go on the wrong treatment paradigm. SpectraCell gives you a chart of treatments that work based on the types of cholesterol you have. According to their data, Statin drugs do NOT work on all types of fats. If a patient comes to me with elevated cholesterol, their doctor will most likely have prescribed a Statin drug. I will recommend we do the Lipoprotein test and base treatment on those results. If the test comes back low risk (very little remnant or low-density LDLs) I may or may not prescribe cholesterol-lowering supplements or medications (because I want to be careful in lowering the cholesterol if hormones are low). Don't forget that hormones are made from cholesterol. In my opinion, it's a balancing act in terms of identifying the right treatment. I always assess risk before I offer treatment. If low density or remnant LDLs are high and antioxidant load is low (low antioxidant diet), then I will immediately treat with wax-matrix niacin no matter the cholesterol levels. If LDL remnant and density particles are not high, then I will analyze diet and lifestyle first and proceed from there.

Treating the Cause with the Power of Belief:

We are taught that we can't lower cholesterol without medication. I teach my patients the opposite.

I have a patient who was concerned about her total cholesterol levels of 360. I told her to focus on exercise, weight loss, and better eating choices and we would re-test her levels every six months. I asked her to believe in her body and she decided to set her mind for success.

As she started to lose weight we saw an initial increase in her cholesterol. I waited six months before I suggested she go off her cholesterol-lowering medication (to give her body time to process the cholesterol). She did and we saw one more increase in her levels, but this was temporary. Her weight had started to decrease in the first few months we were working together, and by year one her cholesterol had finally lowered to just under 300. Six more months of time and her cholesterol lowered to 250. Six more months and we were down to 220.

She believed and put her mind on improving her cholesterol. It did with time, patience, and persistence.

Here is what I have taught my patients to do if they have High Cholesterol:

1. Start by testing Lipoprotein levels to get an idea of the true risk (I like the specialty lab SpectraCell).

2. Exercise.

3. Avoid supplements like Red Yeast Rice because they are no different than a Statin drug (so you may as well use the Statin drug which at least guarantees mechanism and dosing delivery systems whereas supplements are not regulated).

4. Decrease or eliminate foods such as processed sugars and dairy.

5. Increase consumption of antioxidant rich foods (Chapter 5).

6. Use my Pitcher Plant Tincture to help regulate inflammation. See my website for details.

❧ 20 ❧
Irritable Bowel Syndrome (IBS) & GERD (Reflux)

IBS ("leaky gut syndrome") is defined as a "bowel disorder" affecting 24% of women and 19% of men in the United States, accounting for 50% of referrals to gastroenterologists. Patients experience abdominal pain, constipation, and/or diarrhea in the "absence of any other pathology" (www.mdconsult.com/das/pdxmd/body/403746318-10/1411694919?type=med&eid=9-u1.0-_1_mt_1014787). Unfortnately, IBS places patients at high risk for the development of colon cancer.

I class reflux disease (GERD) with IBS, as the two often go hand-in-hand. GERD involves the reflux of gastric juices into the esophagus affecting up to 60% of adults (www.mdconsult.com/das/pdxmd/body/425846255-3/0?type=med&eid=9-u1.0-_1_mt_1014777). The causes and treatments are generally the same with IBS and GERD.

IBS is Diagnosed via:
Abdominal Symptoms such as Pain or Constipation/Diarrhea

Physical Exam

Blood Work (CBC/CMP)

Stool Culture

Colonoscopy

Celiac Disease Screening (Blood Work)

GERD is Diagnosed via:
Endoscopy

Acid Sensation in Chest/Abdomen often with Burping

Conditions associated with IBS/GERD include:
Colitis

Appendicitis

Pancreatitis

Gallbladder Diseases

Menstrual Disorders like Fibroids

Abdominal Infections

Crohn's Disease

Cancer

Fibromyalgia

Obesity

✚ Conventional Medical Treatment Options include:

Pain Medications (i.e. Morphine)

Acid-blocker Medications (i.e. Omeprazole)

Anti-inflammatories (i.e. Ibuprofen)

Surgery

Psychiatric Treatment

Hypnotherapy

Cognitive Behavior

Anti-depressant Medications (i.e. Zoloft)

Laxative medications

Anti-diarrheal Medications (i.e. Loperamide)

Medications to affect Bowel Transit Time (i.e. Lubiprostone, Alosetron)

Reduced Fatty Food Intake

Reduced Caffeine Intake

Antibiotics

✳ Alternative Medical Treatment Options include:

Herbs (i.e. slippery elm)

Hot Packs to Abdomen

Supplements for pain/inflammation (i.e. peppermint oil)

Massage

Probiotics

Acupuncture

✪ Naturopathic Medicine, Treating the Cause of IBS:

According to MDconsult.com, the cause of IBS is "unknown" (www.mdconsult.com/das/pdxmd/body/403746318-10/1411694919?type=med&eid=9-u1.0-_1_mt_1014787), but thought to result from disturbed intestinal mobility and enhanced abdominal sensitivity from problems with seratonin. Seratonin is the neurotransmitter responsible for gut motility and sensation (Chapter 7).

In my opinion, there are many causes of IBS (and GERD): issues with fat metabolism, hormones, toxins, low antioxidant levels, food sensitivities, low glutathione, low seratonin, and negative mind/body connection (Chapters 1-9).

A good place to start in the treatment of IBS and GERD is to look for food sensitivities. I recommend my patients do an elimination diet or a food sensitivity panel to identify specific foods their body doesn't like. An elimination diet involves removal of one food at a time, and for at least three weeks, as it takes time for immune complexes to calm down enough to see a change in symptoms (clinical observation). If the patient does not want to do this, or feels like they have but are still not sure of the foods, then I recommend Immunolabs 154 food test.

Once the food(s) are removed, patients may need other modalities to help heal the gut tissues. I always recommend my patients remove the foods first and add the supplements later: if you don't remove foods first, you will be spinning your wheels with supplements and may or may not ever feel fully well.

I use the following treatments once offending foods are removed:

- Integrative Therapeutics Permeability Factors, 3-6 daily (helps heal the gut lining).

- Slippery Elm Tea *(1 tsp in a cup of hot water is very soothing to sip)*.

- Adrenal herbal support (the adrenals help maintain the intestinal lining, per my clinical experience; I have an IBS formula with adrenal herbs that is very effective in treating the inflammation related to IBS, see my website for details).

- Probiotics.

- 5-HTP (helps build seratonin levels, Chapter 7).

- Glutathione (Chapter 4).

In recent research, glutathione is low in gut tissues of patients with IBS and GERD relative to patients who do not have either condition (Soto et al. 1998). From Chapter 4, glutathione is a detoxification molecule. Foods have toxins in them, especially if you are not eating organically raised, non-GMO (non genetically modified) foods. Constant exposure to toxins could lower glutathione levels in the gut especially in patients who already have a tendency towards a sensitive gut. Adding glutathione does help some patients with IBS/GERD.

I have also found that my Pitcher Plant Formulations (both sublingual and tincture) calm gut inflammation. Some patients, when they first introduce these pitcher plant blends, experience a transient worsening of their symptoms, such as abdominal pain or rectal/vaginal discharge. In Naturopathy, this is called a "healing crisis" whereby things get worse before they get better. I encourage my patients to stay the course if this starts to happen, and usually within one to two months the "healing crisis" has stopped and they are much, much better.

✪ Naturopathic Medicine, Treating the Cause of GERD:

Treatments for GERD are very similar to that which I use for IBS. Food sensitivities and GMO foods are one of the biggest causes of reflux.

The most common foods I see contributing to both conditions include:

Wheat	*Eggs*	*Sugar*
Corn	*Dairy*	

Treating the Cause with the Power of Belief:

I have a patient who initially came to see me for joint pain and I was treating her with acupuncture. As she improved, she no longer needed my services so I did not see her until three years later. This time when she came in she had an array of symptoms, which included fatigue, weakness, abdominal pain, gas, and bloating. I diagnosed her with IBS, hypothyroidism, and adrenal fatigue (Chapter 8). We of course discussed her diet and she decided to start with going off wheat, dairy, and sugar; at the same time, I was working with her to balance out her adrenal and thyroid hormones. I asked that she use some of my herbal formulations to support hormone levels.

I saw her two months later; many of her symptoms had improved (less or no gas/bloating/pain), but the best part was that SHE returned to tell ME that she felt like something was not quite right in the middle part of the day. No matter what she ate over lunch she would get GERD-like symptoms. I thought about it and realized her digestive enzymes may be low, so I recommended she eat a light lunch (maybe soups) and use chewable enzymes. I also had her take a dropperful of my adrenal herbs at the time of day she had symptoms. She came back a few weeks later and reported this made a huge difference.

What really made the difference is that she went from being a victim of her diseases to being empowered: she started to realize when her body was feeling a bit off and brought that concern to me to see if, as a team, we could figure out her deficiency. She listened and her body told her exactly what it needed.

Here is what I have taught my patients to do about IBS/GERD:

1. Eliminate food sensitivities as best as possible.

2. Use glutathione supplementation to support the gut lining (IM or IV is best).

3. Avoid sugar.

4. Avoid GMO foods.

5. Use herbs like slippery elm (as a tea, this is awesome) if an IBS flare starts (if you get exposed to a food you are sensitive to, for example). You can make this tea by stirring into a cup of hot water 1 tsp slippery elm powder. Slippery elm comes in tinctures and capsule forms but this plant's properties are water soluble, so this means it is best as a tea.

6. Use my sublingual glutathione lozenge.

7. Practice stress management. Do things you enjoy and focus on them rather than what is wrong.

8. Use adrenal support. Very few formulas work, so try my formula first to get a baseline. See my website for details.

🙠 21 🙡
Gallbladder Diseases

Your gallbladder is an organ that lies near your liver. Its job is to store bile the liver makes. Bile is released into the gut when you eat a meal, especially a fatty meal. There are different types of gallbladder diseases: cholecystitis is the most common (an infection of the gallbladder). Cholelithiasis is a gallstone. Annually, 0.6% of Americans experience an inflamed gallbladder, while stones affect up to 30% of Americans (www.mdconsult.com/das/pdxmd/body/403746318-8/1411689153type=med&eid =9-u1.0-_1_mt_1014767). Symptoms of gallbladder disease include abdominal pain, nausea, vomiting, fever, chills, or lack of appetite.

The Gallbladder Diseases are Diagnosed via:
Physical Exam
Ultrasound
Blood Work (CBC/WBC count)

**The following conditions tend to be associated
with Gallbladder Diseases:**
Liver Disease
IBS
Menopause
Perimenopause
Obesity
Pregnancy
Oral Birth Control Use

✚ Conventional Medical Treatment Options include:
Medications (i.e. NSAIDs)
Surgery
Weight Loss

✳ Alternative Medical Treatment Options include:
Herbs
Hot Lemon/Water Will Help to Stimulate the Liver
Enzymes (Pancreatic or Plant)
Gallbladder Support Supplements

✺ Naturopathic Medicine, Treating the Cause:

Gallbladder issues are usually a result of inflammation (Chapter 6) settling in from food sensitivities (clinical observation), which essentially is IBS (Chapter 20).

If you have the gallbladder removed, it does not mean your symptoms will go away. You may feel good initially, but the problem hurting the gallbladder will still be there.

To Nourish the Gallbladder:

• Remove foods you are sensitive to. Eggs seem to create the most problems for the gallbladder.

• Do castor oil packs on your liver/gallbladder (Chapter 35).

• Use liver support herbs (i.e. dandelion, milk thistle) AFTER or AS the offending food(s) are removed. If you don't, symptoms may persist despite the best herbs/supplements. I have a blend I use called Immune Formula (www.goweyresearchgroup.com) that has a high percentage of liver support herbs. I use this formula for both liver and immune system support while patients are coming off the foods their body doesn't like (eggs usually).

I also help my patients consider whether or not they should go off birth control pills and hormone replacement. Hormones (especially oral estrogen) may be a cause of gallbladder symptoms.

From a Blog I posted to my website on 12/31/12:

Most women (and men) are put on hormones for menopause or andropause. Symptoms patients present with include hot flashes, fatigue, insomnia, depression, anxiety, loss or gain in weight, or mood swings. Physicians will run the hormone levels and then decide on a course of treatment that involves the use of prescription hormones; the goal of these treatments is to keep levels at "reproductive age" normals. When patients go on these hormones, they often feel better initially, but over time may actually end up having more problems.

A patient came to my office with chronic abdominal pain, which had recently led to the removal of her gallbladder. After surgical removal of the gallbladder, she was still having a great deal of abdominal pains. She was also having a difficult time losing weight. Upon taking her case, I learned that she had been on an oral dose of estrogen for several years, and over that time her abdominal symptoms had been worsening as had the weight gain. I was suspicious that she was struggling with metabolizing the estrogen (which is very common), and that those symptoms of estrogen excess were harming her gallbladder. Upon taking her off the estrogen, I had her do castor oil packs over her liver (Chapter 35), supported her liver with a few teaspoons of my Immune Support herbs daily, worked with her to make sure none of her other hormones were off (she was slightly hypothyroid) and within a month the abdominal pains were gone. She also started to lose some weight.

I find that the gallbladder is relatively easy to treat. Once you identify what is aggravating it and treat the cause, the gallbladder bounces back quickly. I do not see a need for most gallbladder surgeries.

Treating the Cause with the Power of Belief:

I had a new patient come to my practice with extreme chronic abdominal pain. After I looked at his records I determined IBS was the underlying cause of his symptoms: the resultant inflammation from the IBS had extended to his gallbladder and liver. He was concerned of the long-term effects of the IBS on his gallbladder. He also thought the gallbladder inflammation would be permanent, but I assured him that if he worked at it the inflammation would and could decrease.

He dug his heels in and decided to listen to his body in terms of the foods that were safe for him to eat; he pulled processed sugar out of his diet and started to use herbs as needed to support both his liver and gallbladder (he used my Immune Formula). After a few weeks he was very stable and the abdominal pain was gone!

Here is what I have taught my patients to do if they have Gallbladder Issues:

1. Use bitters such as watercress or dandelion leaves to stimulate the release of bile from the liver and gallbladder. As soon as you taste something bitter, bile is released. The important thing is to TASTE the bitters and not just use them as a supplement you swallow.

2. Use castor oil packs over the liver/gallbladder if you are experiencing acute pain, OR you may do the packs as preventative medicine (Chapter 35).

3. Try to avoid eating eggs. Eggs and the gallbladder don't seem to mix (clinical observation).

4. Keep hormones in balance. Too high of estrogen can create problems for the gallbladder.

✌ 22 ✎
Chronic Kidney Stones

Kidney stones are defined as the abnormal deposit of minerals (calcium primarily) in the kidneys. The body may occasionally pass these stones into the urinary tract, causing pain: 12% of men and 6% of women form stones, with the cause generally cited as "idiopathic", meaning there is no "identifiable cause" (www.mdconsult.com/das/pdxmd/body/406922261-3/1424647993?type=med&eid=9-u1.0-_1_mt_1014832). While most stones are calcium oxalate or phosphate, some can be formed from uric acid, struvite, or cystine.

Stones are Diagnosed via:
Kidney Ultrasound

Urinalysis

PTH Level Analysis

Pyelogram

Stone Analysis (to identify type)

✚ Conventional Medical Treatment Options include:
Lithotripsy

Pain Medications (i.e. Morphine)

Anti-inflammatory Medications (i.e. NSAIDs)

Calcium Blocker Medications (i.e. Nifedipine)

Mineral Balance Medications (i.e. Diuretics)

Uric Acid Blockers (i.e. Allopurinol)

Increased Water Intake

Diet Changes (i.e. Less Protein)

✳ Alternative Medical Treatment Options include:
Apple Cider Vinegar

Herbs

Calcium/Magnesium/Potassium Supplements

Vitamin D

❂ Naturopathic Medicine, Treating the Cause:
Kidney stones often result from problems with vitamin and mineral metabolism, inflammation, or low antioxidant levels (Chapters 2, 3, 5, and 6).

I had a patient who had been struggling with stones for 18 years. She had her first when pregnant with her son. Recently the frequency of the stones increased annually to every six months. Imaging studies showed that her kidneys looked like cauliflower because there were so many stone deposits.

She also had experienced multiple tendon and ligament ruptures, which made me think she had trouble metabolizing calcium (calcium is used as a building block/strengthener in connective tissue) while Vitamin D is used to absorb calcium. Her blood work showed her vitamin D was actually quite low.

Chronic kidney stones are associated with increased oxidative (low antioxidant) damage: new stones contribute to further stone formation via oxidative damage to the kidneys (Carrasco-Valiente et al. 2012 and Meimaridou et al. 2006). Acidic body pH accelerates this process. This was part of my recommendations to her:

- Increase pH to more alkaline. You can test your urine pH with Litmus test strips. Urine pH should be around 6.5-7; under 5 or 6 and you are running too acidic; over 7-7.5 and you are too alkaline. Your body uses minerals such as calcium out of your bones to keep your pH normal at 7.4.

- Increase antioxidant intake via berries/colorful veggies.

- Take Thorne Vitamin D 5000 units one daily (this product I have seen absorbs well as shown by pre and post patient labs). Putting patients on Vitamin D is actually very controversial, but every patient I have seen with stone issues has a vitamin D issue as well, and when I put them on a good one they see an improvement in how they feel.

After a few months, a repeat x-ray did not show any stones in her left kidney, a first for her in years. She also had a significant reduction of them in her right kidney.

Treating the Cause with the Power of Belief:

The patient I talked about in this chapter believed strongly that Naturopathic Medicine would heal her. She drove three hours from another city to see me and made all the changes I suggested. She believed!

Here is what I have taught my patients to do if they have Kidney Stones:

1. Keep protein balanced in the diet; too much protein contributes to the development of stones.

2. Too little Vitamin D contributes to the development of stones, but too much can as well. Just a little absorbable Vitamin D a day is fine. Thorne

makes a fantastic one that is 5000 IUs.

3. Take care of the liver; if the liver is unhappy it can reflect on the kidneys and vice versa.

23
Thyroid Diseases

The thyroid is susceptible to the development of several different types of diseases. The most common are hypothyroidism, hyperthyroidism, and Hashimoto's hypothyroidism.

Hypothyroidism is the decreased production of thyroid hormones by the thyroid gland. Hyperthyroidism is the increased production of thyroid hormones by the thyroid gland. Hashimoto's is a type of autoimmune hypothyroidism whereby antibodies actually attack the thyroid gland.

Hypothyroidism (including Hashimoto's) and hyperthyroidism can have some similarity in symptoms. Patients with these diseases may notice changes to weight or mood. However, patients with hyperthyroidism usually experience increased appetite, increased heart rate, and decreased weight. Hypothyroid patients tend to gain weight and may notice adverse changes to hair, skin, or nails.

Overall in United States, hypothyroidism affects more women than men at a rate of 10:1. Hashimoto's is the most common type of hypothyroidism (www.mdconsult.com/das/pdxmd/body/403903122-6/1412398866?type=med&eid=9-u1.0-_1_mt_1014742).

Thyroid Disorders are Diagnosed via:
Physical Exam/History
Blood Work (TSH/T4/T3)
Anti-TPO Antibodies (to Identify Hashimoto's)

Disorders associated with Thyroid Problems include:
Fibromyalgia
Menstrual Irregularities
Unexplained Weight Gain or Loss
Sleep Disturbances
Chronic Fatigue
Other Autoimmune Diseases
Arthritis
Depression
Anxiety

✚ Conventional Medical Treatment Options include:

Thyroid Medication

Surgical Removal of Thyroid

Thyroid Ablation

✳ Alternative Medical Treatment Options include:

Herbs

Supplements (i.e. Thyroid Support)

Mineral and Vitamins

Reiki

✪ Naturopathic Medicine, Treating the Cause:

The thyroid is very sensitive to vitamin and mineral imbalances (Chapters 2-3), inflammation (Chapter 6), and toxins (Chapter 4-5).

For example, Hashimoto's is characterized by fluctuating levels of thyroid stimulating hormone (TSH): one week the TSH may be low, but then it may be high. Patients with this disease may see a rapid change in symptoms, from low to high mood, to weight gain or loss, to appetite gain or loss. In my quest to help patients with Hashimoto's, I have found inflammation (body-wide), environmental toxins, adrenal fatigue, and digestive problems (i.e. food sensitivities, especially wheat) contributing to the thyroid's rapidly changing TSH. In addition, my colleague Dr. Friedman, NMD has found low Vitamin D to be a contributing factor (Friedman 2013).

I approach thyroid disease different in every patient because these conditions can be tricky to treat, no matter the type. I suggest working closely with your Naturopath to identify what is causing problems for your thyroid.

Hashimoto's Disease:

- Remove offending foods/sensitivities.
- Reduce sugar intake.
- Look at possible environmental toxin exposures.
- Use herbs to modulate (reduce) inflammation.
- Keep gut tissue as healthy as possible.

Hypothyroidism:

- Consume foods with supportive nutrients for the thyroid, i.e. kelp (thyroid needs iodine to make hormones).
- Increase selenium/zinc via Brazil nuts or supplementation (these are needed to make T4 into usable T3).
- Manage stress levels.

- Treat any adrenal fatigue (my Adrenal Herbs work great).
- Use medications if necessary.

Hyperthyroidism:

- Identify what is causing thyroid to overproduce hormones. I often see a gut disorder doing this, such as IBS.
- Use medications if necessary.

Treating the Cause with the Power of Belief:

I have a patient who always knows when her thyroid is "not right", but this knowledge only came about after months of my encouraging and supporting her in listening to her body. As a physician, if you encourage your patients to listen to their bodies and honor what it is telling them you make leaps and bounds ahead in terms of the prevention of disease. This particular patient always knows when it is time to check her labs and she lets me know when she feels we need to change medication doses.

Here is what I have taught my patients to do if they have Thyroid Disorders:

1. Nourish the thyroid with foods such as seaweed products (they have healthy but not toxic levels of iodine).

2. Take care of the adrenal glands (Chapter 8) because it communicates with the thyroid; if something is wrong with one gland, it will reflect on the other.

3. Be careful of environmental exposures. The thyroid is very sensitive to pollutants such as radiation and heavy metals.

4. Avoid gluten-containing foods. Gluten bothers the gut, which in turn aggravates the thyroid (clinical observation).

❧ 24 ❧
Dysmenorrhea
(Painful Menstrual Cramps)
& PMS

Most women have experienced or do experience pain (dysmenorrhea) with their menstrual cycle. Dysmenorrhea affects 90% of female adolescents and 50% of adults. Of these, 15% of women experience pain so severe that work and activities become adversely affected (www.mdconsult.com/das/pdxmd/body/403746318-14/1411704308?-type=med&eid=9-u1.0-_1_mt_1014318). PMS (pre-menstrual symptoms) is defined as symptoms in the days before the cycle starts such as irritability, bloating, breast tenderness, fatigue, headaches, moodiness, or depression (www.mdconsult.com/das/pdxmd/body/436693809-3/1504168633?type=med&eid=9-u1.0-_1_mt_1014339).

Painful Menstrual Cramps are Diagnosed via:
Ultrasound
Clinical History Taking
Physical Exam
Blood Work
Exploratory Laparoscopy
Pregnancy Test
Urinalysis

Conditions associated with
Painful Menstrual Cramps include:
Pelvic Inflammatory Disease
IUD Use
Ovarian Cysts
Uterine Fibroids
Endometriosis
IBS
Fibromyalgia
Cancer
PMS is Diagnosed via:
History

Conditions often associated with PMS include:
IBS

Bipolar Disorder

Thyroid Disorders

Fibroids

Ovarian Cyst

Uterine Fibroids

Infertility

Endometriosis

MS

Fibromyalgia

✚ Conventional Medical Treatment Options include:
Birth Control Pills

Laparoscopic surgery (if PMS is linked to endometriosis/fibroids/cysts)

Hysterectomy

Anti-depressant Medications (i.e. Prozac)

Smoking/Alcohol Cessation

✳ Alternative Medical Treatment Options include:
Acupuncture

Massage

Omega Oils

Herbs

Calcium/Magnesium Supplements

◑ Naturopathic Medicine, Treating the Cause:
Your menstrual cycle is divided into two phases: follicular and luteal. Follicular phase occurs in the first half of the monthly cycle starting with the day that you menstruate and generally goes to day 14. The second half of your cycle goes from day 14 to about 24-31 and involves the building of the uterine lining. The purpose of the building of the lining is to maintain a fertilized follicle should you become pregnant. If you do not become pregnant, this lining is shed when you start your menstrual cycle.

Unfortunately, it is the luteal phase that creates a lot of adverse symptoms such as depression, anxiety, bloating, breast pain, headache, fatigue, mood swings, decreased libido, insomnia, weight gain, or migraines. In my experience, signaling molecules (the ping-pong balls/Internet signal, Chapter 6), such as prostaglandins, are overactive in women with menstrual pain. This over activity of the immune system creates inflammation that then creates the symptoms.

Factors that contribute to the inflammation include:

Food Sensitivities

Low Glutathione Levels (Chapter 4)

Low Vitamin/Mineral Levels (Chapters 2-3)

Low Omega Oils (Chapter 1)

Disruption in Meridian Flow (belly button rings for example can cause painful cramps/PMS because they block the acupuncture point Ren 8)

Processed Sugar in Diet

Underlying Conditions such as Fibroids/Cysts/Endometriosis

Cancer

Poor Liver Function

To illustrate how I work through identifying the cause of PMS and painful cramps, I thought it might be easiest to present a patient case.

Patient Case:

At 15, this woman developed very painful menstrual cramps with extreme PMS. Her PMS was characterized by low mood for two weeks before her cycle started. She also experienced irritability, bloating (abdominal), breast tenderness, body aches, eczema, hot flashes, and insomnia. She would cry frequently and often. When the menstrual bleeding started, she would have intense cramps that would last for three days and be so bad she would vomit. She would not be able to go to school or work.

After suffering with this for 10 years, she came to see me. I started with testing her for Celiac disease. Celiac disease is autoimmune gluten intolerance and is a cause of inflammation. She tested positive for it, so I had her eliminate wheat/gluten from her diet. Within three days of a gluten-free diet she noticed positive changes to both her skin and mood. Two months later her cycle was less painful and she had less bloating, irritability, and moodiness.

As she improved (by not eating gluten) I added some vitamins/minerals (i.e. magnesium) and Omega oils (Chapter 1) which also helped decrease cramps. I added my Immune Formula for liver support. This formulation she described as "making me feel very even-tempered". I usually add herbs once we have identified the "Obstacle to Cure" (Hannheman 1921), which is the one thing(s) that most prevents a patient from improving. In this case, her Obstacle was wheat *and I added supplements later. I did not use the supplements to treat the diseases, only to support her body.*

Treating the Cause with the Power of Belief:

For women, symptoms surrounding the menstrual cycle always show that something in the body is out of balance.

A recent new patient came to me saying, "I just know my body is out of whack." Now this is my type of patient! Someone who knows their health is not quite where it should be and wants help figuring out their Obstacles. I love it!

After a few months of working together, she was on a good road to "wellness". But it all started because she believed!

**Here is what I have taught my patients to do
if they struggle with their Cycles:**

1. The liver is the master of the menstrual cycle. Happy liver=happy cycle.

2. Get acupuncture regularly. It helps keep the liver in balance, which is key for a healthy cycle.

3. Avoid processed sugar. Not good for the liver. Processed foods and sugar in the diet seems to make women feel angry or short-tempered. If you don't believe me, go give a piece of cake with lots of frosting to a woman going through PMS and watch her behavior for the next hour.

4. My Immune Herbs are largely liver support hormones. These are fantastic for keeping the liver in balance, especially if sugar is avoided.

5. My Pitcher Plant Formulas are amazing for lowering the ping-pong ball/ Internet signaling process (Chapter 6) as it relates to the menstrual cycle. Make these herbs part of the treatment protocol. I have found the Pitcher Plant lowers fibrinogen, an inflammatory marker made by the liver.

✏ 25 ✏
Abnormal Pap Smears (Cervical Dysplasia)

Cervical dysplasia is defined as "pre-cancerous" cells on a cervix, and is identified via the Pap. If left untreated, this condition may lead to cervical cancer. Most women do not have symptoms. If the Pap smear comes back as abnormal, your gynecologist will do a biopsy to see if the abnormality has gone into deeper tissues. The Pap smear has reduced the rate of cervical cancer by 90%, but there are still 12,900 new cases and 4,400 deaths annually (www.mdconsult.com/das/pdxmd/body/403903122-5/14-12397058type=med&eid=9-u1.0-_1_mt_1014649).

Cervical Dysplasia/Cancer is Diagnosed via:
Pap Smear

Colposcopy (Biopsy)

Ultrasound/CT Scan/PET Scan if Pathology has Progressed

Diseases associated with Cervical Dysplasia include:
Immune Disorders

Malnutrition

Hormonal Disorders

Fibromyalgia

IBS

Patients often ask me if they should do the biopsy (colposcopy) if the Pap came back as abnormal. Pap Smears are not 100% accurate, so the biopsy is used to confirm the Pap diagnosis. The biopsy also helps determine whether or not the pathology has gone deeper into the cervix. I do recommend patients follow the standard of care and have the biopsy done if their Pap results come back LSIL or HSIL (mild to advanced dysplasia). Since the time I published my first book, *Your Cervix (Just) Has a Cold*, I have found West Coast Pathology Labs, a company that has specific Pap testing that can look to see if you have the genetics (called Oncogenes) for the development of cervical cancer. They can also test for the exact type of HPV you may have.

✚ Conventional Medical Treatment Options include:
Hysterectomy

LEEP/Cryosurgery

Watch and Wait

Biopsy Removal of Damaged Tissue

Chemo/Radiation

Smoking Cessation

Vaccine to HPV

Condom Use

✳ **Alternative Medical Treatment Options include:**

Herbs

Supplements such as Folic Acid

◉ **Naturopathic Medicine, Treating the Cause:**

HPV is a virus that is blamed for causing abnormal Pap results, but anything that stimulates inflammation is a major contributor. I do not think HPV is the ultimate cause of cervical dysplasia: the virus becomes active (becomes a cause) only if the cervical cells themselves are not healthy (Gowey 2014).

I have found the following factors allow HPV to become active:

Poor nutrition (i.e. Low Antioxidant Levels)

Processed Sugars in Diet

Food Sensitivities

Environmental Toxin Exposure

Cigarette Smoking

Alcohol Consumption

Excess Estrogen

Birth Control Pills

Hormone Replacement Therapy

I do a combination of treatments for this disease. Please read *Your Cervix (Just) Has a Cold* for more details.

My colleague Sherry Tackett, Women's Health Nurse Practitioner, feels that the HPV vaccine is giving women cervical dysplasia. Girls who had the vaccination series for HPV, who have had a history of normal Paps and no HPV, are showing abnormal Paps and HPV (shortly after receiving the vaccination).

I am not against vaccinations; I am for good medicine. I do not feel the HPV vaccine is good medicine because it was introduced to the market with very limited testing.

Some vaccinations are now showing a link to causing cancer (www.CDC.org), such as the polio vaccine. The CDC posted briefly on their site a study that has shown the polio vaccination caused cancer. This link was pulled quickly off their site, but not quick enough. One of my patients saw it and posted it on her Facebook page, which is how I found out.

The other aspect to consider with the HPV vaccine is that it is only a few strands of a virus that is dozens and dozens of strands. Just because you protect yourself against one or two doesn't protect you against the others. You will still need to use protection.

And remember, from my perspective, it is more important to treat the reason a virus may be active and not the virus itself.

Treating the Cause with the Power of Belief:

From one of my patients:

I was diagnosed with HPV (Human Papilloma Virus) at the age of 20. I had no knowledge of the virus prior to the diagnosis. I thought my world was coming to an end. I was certain that this was going to be the way I would die. My life completely fell apart in the matter of one appointment with the gynecologist.

After the diagnosis, I was passed to a new doctor in the same office, one who was said to have more experience with women who were dealing with this virus. After two surgeries and several treatments, it was apparent that I needed someone who was more equipped to help me. So I was once again passed on to another doctor.

The new doctor was supposedly a specialist. He was one of few gynocologists in the Phoenix area. So I paid him a visit. I was told that Aldera would be the miracle treatment. Aldera is a topical cream that burns the top layer of skin slowly. The idea is that the Aldera will eat away the top layers of skin until eventually the dysplasia (or precancerous cells)/condyloma (commonly known as warts) is no longer noticeable.

I was told by the doctor that if the treatments with Aldera didn't work, my only other option would be a vulvectomy. This is where they remove the vulva, clitoris, and labia. A terrifying thought for a young girl just starting adulthood.

After seeing the specialist regularly for about a year, he became very ill and closed his practice. I was once again passed along to a new doctor. Nothing changed with her. Everything she had told me I had already heard from every other doctor and specialist I had seen. There was no new news and there seemed to be no hope.

After seeing her for about two years, I started to give up hope. I had not seen any results from the countless treatments and four surgeries. My condition had not improved the slightest since the initial diagnosis.

After several years, I began to accept this virus and even went as far as to make it part of my identity. I was now the girl with HPV. It was no longer just HPV. I started to address it as "my HPV".

I began my life as a sick and hopeless young girl. One who would never find love, one who would never find peace, one who would never find hope, and one who would never find good health. I became a very hopeless person.

But after a while, I decided to pull out of it. I wanted to believe that I was something more. I desired to create a new identity.

I started searching for a new doctor, one who would help me to really understand what I was up against, one who could educate me on how this virus is really affecting my body and most importantly, how could I treat this effectively.

I was blessed to have Dr. Gowey come into my life. I have learned so much from her. She has taught me how to listen to my body and how to start teaching my body to heal itself. While being monitored by Dr. Gowey, I have made some serious changes to my lifestyle. I have changed everything from diet, to exercise, to my whole paradigm. My immune system finally started to respond and attack the virus. I was more than excited to hear the news. This was the best news I had heard since the initial diagnosis. Although my immune system started to have an effective response to the different changes I had been making, I still knew there was something more that needed to happen.

After several months of racking my brain as to what needed to change, the answer hit me like a ton of bricks. I'm holding onto the virus. I realized that I am physically holding on to this virus, and keeping myself ill. "Why would someone do that?" Is the question I had to ask. The answer is actually very simple. I have been using this virus as a guard. I am afraid of rejection and afraid of love. I can use this virus as an excuse to not allow myself to become vulnerable.

After really understanding why I harbored this virus and how it benefits me, I have decided to take a different route. I am no longer claiming this virus. It is no longer part of my identity and I am finally ready to move on with my life and allow myself to become vulnerable. It's in vulnerability that we are really able to heal. When we allow ourselves to be vulnerable, there is no longer a battle within. We are at peace, and we can heal. There are remedies out there to help *speed up the process, but before any remedy can start to help us we have to stop the internal battle.* — ER, Phoenix, AZ

**Here is what I have taught my patients to do
if they have Cervical Dysplasia:**

1. Identify the Obstacle.

2. Read the book *Your Cervix (Just) Has a Cold* to help you identify Obstacles.

3. Use the Gowey Protocol® Gel via vaginal insertion (as a prescription; your physician can call in to compounding pharmacies or you can get it from my office).

4. Stay positive. You can kick this.

❧ 26 ❧
Symptomatic Menopause

Menopause is diagnosed as the cessation of the menstrual cycle for at least 12 months. Symptoms include vaginal atrophy, hot flashes, pain with intercourse, mood changes, skin atrophy, or chronic urinary tract infections. Menopause may come about naturally or may be induced surgically via hysterectomy.

Menopause is Diagnosed via:
Clinical Diagnosis through History Taking
FSH Levels (Increased in Menopause)
Low Estrogen/Progesterone/Testosterone

Menopause is a normal function of aging and is not generally associated with other medical conditions, unless the woman has had a hysterectomy (surgically induced menopause); however, early menopause may be associated with conditions such as:

Cardiovascular Disease
Osteoporosis
Osteoarthritis
Chronic Urinary Tract Infections
Type II Diabetes
Cancer Chemotherapy (www.mdconsult.com/das/pdxmd/
body/4039031224/1412396832?type=med&eid=9-u1.0-_1_mt_1014332)

✚ **Conventional Medical Treatment Options include**
Hormone Replacement Therapy
Anti-depressant Medications (i.e. Zoloft)
High Blood Pressure Medications (i.e. Clonidine, Gabapentin)

✳ **Alternative Medical Treatment Options include:**
Vitamin E
Phytoestrogens
Herbs (i.e. Dong Quai, Black Cohosh, Vitex)
Calcium/Vitamin D
Herb-based Hormones (i.e. Health Food Store Purchased Progesterone)

✪ **Naturopathic Medicine, Treating the Cause:**
Symptoms from menopause come from anything causing inflammation (Chapter 6)

either in the gut or liver (clinical experience).

I find that liver herbs are key for use in treating hot flashes. I explain to my patients that a change in hormones energetically changes the way the liver metabolizes (my theory). Herbs work best synergized with other herbs; my Immune Formula is a combination of liver and immune herbs and is an example. I actually use this formula for treating menopausal hot flashes, as it is very nourishing to the liver. A lot of people use milk thistle to treat the liver, but I rarely prescribe herbs in isolation.

Taking sugar and alcohol out of the diet is also important if a patient is having hot flashes. Sugar is very hard on liver metabolism (clinical observation).

I do the following to work with women who have hot flashes (I focus on treating the liver):

Acupuncture

Remove Processed Sugars

Liver Support Herbs

Castor Oil Packs (Chapter 35)

Homeopathy

I have found bioidentical hormones are necessary only if hormone levels are extremely low and unbalanced relative to each other (i.e. low estrogen with high testosterone). The patient may need some estrogen for a while to regain balance. Be careful with hormones, however. I am learning at cancer conferences that there are significant correlations between the ingestion of hormones and breast cancer (OncANP Conference July 2013).

Treating the Cause with the Power of Belief:

While most women know when they are going through menopause because of the symptoms that start (such as hot flashes), my patients know when they get hot flashes they have done something that put their system out of balance. They will tell ME what they did that caused the symptoms. And they always know what did it (i.e. sugar, alcohol, not enough exercise, a food they are sensitive to, they stopped their herbs), and then they will quickly go back to putting their body and life into balance.

Here is what I have taught my patients to do if they struggle with symptoms due to Menopause:

1. Avoid processed sugars.

2. Get weekly acupuncture.

3. Use castor oils packs (Chapter 35).

4. My Immune Formula is very useful for supporting liver functions.

5. Bioidentical hormones may or may not be necessary when going through perimenopause or menopause if you work to identify your Obstacles.

27
Pain from Joint or Spine Diseases

Pain is subjective. It is difficult for a physician to accurately judge the level of pain patients are in from spine or joint diseases because everyone experiences pain differently.

Spine and Joint Diseases are Diagnosed via:
Physical Exam
X-ray
MRI or CT Scan
Labs such as SED or CRP to test for inflammation

They can be associated with any number of medical conditions including:
Depression
Fibromyalgia
Menstrual Pain
Nutritional Deficiencies
IBS
Gallbladder Problems

✚ **Conventional Medical Treatment Options include:**
Anti-inflammatory Medications (i.e. Ibuprofen)
Pain Medications (i.e. Morphine)
Muscle Relaxers (i.e. Soma)
Surgery (i.e. Fusions)
Steroid Shots
Physical Therapy
Medical Marijuana

✳ **Alternative Medical Treatment Options include:**
Herbs such as *Aconitum* or *Gelsemium* in LOW doses (only use these herbs if monitored by your Naturopathic Physician as they contain alkaloids that can cause excess sedation if not monitored properly, DiPasquale 2009)
Herbal Anti-inflammatories
Massage
Acupuncture
Medical Marijuana

❂ Naturopathic Medicine, Treating the Cause:

Pain comes from problems within the immune and nervous systems (Chapters 6-7). Recent research has shown that cells from the nervous system (called glial cells) communicate with the immune system cells when something is not right. This message then goes back to the glial cells. The signal will continue to bounce back and forth (Txekova et al. 2014), contributing to the sensation of pain.

Dr. David A. Tallman, DC, NMD is a specialist in supporting the body's ability to heal from disorders that cause chronic pain, such as spine diseases. Please refer to his website www.arizonaprolotherapy.com for pre and post MRI images from patients with degenerative diseases he has treated.

Here is one of Dr. Tallman's articles on spine disorders, published in *Naturopathic Doctor News and Reviews* in November 2012:

The spinal disc allows vertebrates to enjoy an incredible amount of freedom of movement. This freedom of movement can become greatly hampered when the disc becomes adversely affected. Spinal disc disorders (SDDs) are an extremely common pathology, likely to affect nearly everyone if they live long enough. SDDs are a massive burden to the population and economy, costing untold amounts of money and production loss.

The spinal disc is often the punished bystander to paraspinal ligament injury. I have found with treating thousands of SDD patients, that many of them have been subjected to motor vehicle crashes or similar traumas at some point in their life. When I take a history, I am very careful to ask about vehicular collisions. I have many patients casually deny that they have been involved in a car crash until I ask them to look back into the distant past. I then often hear the, "Oh yeah, I was in a roll-over in the 1970s," or "Do you mean that crash many years ago when a semi-trailer totaled my car and the Jaws of Life pried me out?"...after the dust settles, the spinal discs are often left in a hostile environment due to permanent ligament damage that holds the discs in place. Paraspinal ligament damage places the annular fibers in a hypermobile environment. What appears to be a spinal hypomobility due to muscle guarding is, in reality, a hypermobility. The body reacts to the spinal hypermobility by the slow process of vertebral fusion, radiographically identified by vertebral body spurs, facet enlargement, and ligamentum flavum hypertrophy.

Acute low back pain cases have a positive correlation with annular tears and disc bulges...patients presenting at hospitals with acute, severe low back pain always had annular tears, and 87% of them had disc bulges...In my opinion, having a disc bulge, disc desiccation, or facet hypertrophy should not be considered a "normal" process of aging, as there is always an underlying cause when there is a deviation from one's genetic potential. Everyone's perception of pain is different. I have treated many patients with very minor bulges suffering tremendous pain and have seen severe extrusions cause comparatively minimal discomfort. It is my opinion that most of the pain associated with SDDs is actually muscular in origin, as the paraspinal muscles attempt to perform the task originally delegated to the ligaments. Once the ligament issue is corrected, most pain associated with SDDs will diminish, even in severely desiccated or extruded discs.

Case Study:

A patient presented to my office with low back pain of over two years' duration. She had a recent lumbar magnetic resonance (MR) scan that demonstrated a severe disc bulge at L5-S1 and L4-5. Her history included injuring her back while carrying a heavy mattress upstairs two years prior to her first visit. She remembers hearing a popping sound and immediately suffering severe low back pain...since this injury. She reported undergoing physical therapy and the obligatory epidural cortisone shots that did not help her symptoms. She also received chiropractic care and acupuncture that afforded her temporary symptom relief. The patient reported that her daily symptoms included constant low back pain with...occasional urinary incontinence, an inability to walk for appreciable distances, and worst of all, according to the patient, an inability to pick up her grandchild without pain. She presented to my office after being evaluated by an orthopedic spine surgeon who recommended immediate decompression, laminectomy, and fusion of L4-5.

After performing an orthopedic and MR film evaluation, I informed the patient that a referral to a surgeon was imminent if her symptoms did not improve. I recommended a course of precision treatments with prolotherapy to the facet capsules, interspinous, supraspinous, and intertransverse ligaments from L3 to S1. I deposited proliferants with a specialized direct needling technique to the aforementioned ligaments. She was treated every 5 weeks for 5 sessions, followed by 3 more treatments every 8 weeks. Her global symptoms improved with every visit with regard to pain-free range of motion, radiation of pain, and myospasms. Her urinary incontinence also abated after a few treatments. She was most pleased by being able to hold and carry her grandchild without suffering painful consequences. A follow-up MRI scan was performed to reevaluate her discs.

Basically, his article is saying that the patient experienced relief from pain by treating ligaments.

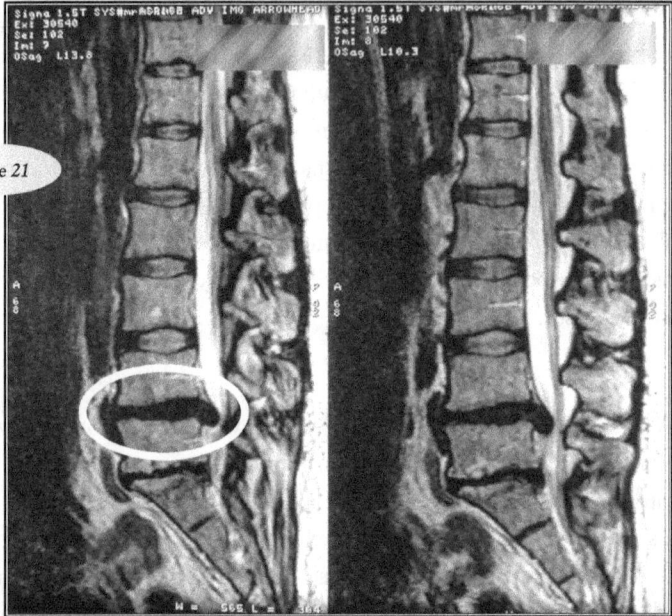

Figure 21

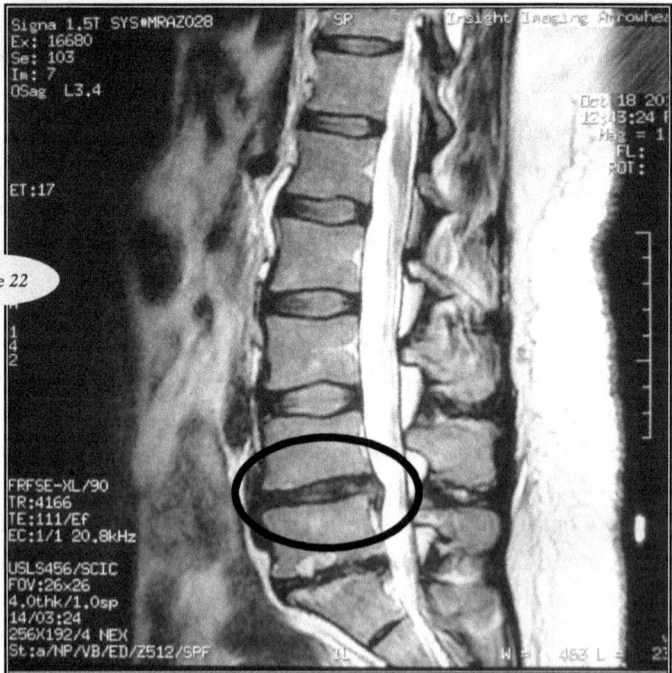

Figure 22

Figures 21 and 22. The herniated disc is circled in the pre- (Figure 21) and post- (Figure 22) treatment MRIs from this particular case.

Treating the Cause with the Power of Belief:

I have a patient with extensive osteoarthritic joint disease affecting his neck, low back, knees, and shoulders. He is in constant pain, or at least he was until we started working together.

When I first met him, he was eating lots of wheat/grains, dairy, and sugar! It took some convincing, but I told him I was noticing other patients experience some pain relief when they took foods that promoted inflammation out of their diet. He decided to give it a try by pulling out diary first and lowering his intake of processed sugars.

He gave this a few months and then came to see me after a trip home to visit family (during which he ate a lot of the foods he had been pulling out).

Here are his words:

Well doc, I allowed myself to be like everyone else at Thanksgiving. I ate sugar. I ate dairy. Dairy gave me a rash on my arms that itched like mad and the sugar made my neck hurt bad. I don't want either anymore. My body is ok as long as I don't eat those things.

My patients know their bodies! They believe!

Here is what I have taught my patients to do
for Osteoarthritic Pain:

1. See Dr. Tallman for prolotherapy or other joint-building treatments (arizonaprolotherapy.com).

2. Go off foods that tend to aggravate joints/inflammation: dairy, wheat, and sugar are the worst.

3. Learn to love yoga.

4. Rest more often, give the joints a rest.

5. Stretch in the morning.

6. Do acupuncture/cold laser treatments.

7. Keep mineral levels good, i.e. use a magnesium/trace mineral supplement (liquid is great!).

8. Treat other underlying conditions, i.e. IBS can create joint pain because it lowers absorption of nutrients.

9.   Pitcher plant castor oil packs. (See www.goweyresearchgroup.com) Rub the oil on the painful area, then apply a hot water bottle wrapped in a cloth. Rest 10-15 minutes. This helps lower inflammation and muscle spasms.

10. Avoid eating processed sugars!

❧ 28 ❧
Fibromyalgia

Fibromyalgia is defined as a "chronic musculoskeletal disorder" with pain in locations on the body called tender points (www.mdconsult.com/das/pdxmd/body/403903122-7/1412401531?type=med&eid=9-u1.0-_1_mt_1014924). It is usually diagnosed in the absence of any other pathology (meaning no other pain syndrome can be identified).

Fibromyalgia is Diagnosed via:
Good History Taking on Symptoms
11 out of 18 Tender Points with Sensitivity
Elimination of Other Medical Conditions
Labs (Sed Rate/Thyroid Panel/CBC/RF/CK/LV FunctionTests)

Conditions often associated with Fibromyalgia include:
Cardiovascular disease
IBS
Depression
Fatigue
Osteoarthritis
Sleep Disorders
Cancer

✚ Conventional Medical Treatment Options include:
Sleep
Anti-depressants (i.e. Amitryptyline)
Pain Medications (i.e. Oxycodone, Morphine)
Muscle Relaxers (i.e. Soma)
Anti-inflammatories
Synthetic Cannabinoids (i.e. Nabilone)
Medical Marijuana

✳ Alternative Medical Treatment Options include:
Herbs (i.e. Medical Marijuana)
Diet Changes
Massage

Acupuncture

Mineral Supplements (i.e. Magnesium)

Sleep

✪ Naturopathic Medicine, Treating the Cause:

Fibromyalgia is actually a very controversial diagnosis (http://www.mdconsult.com/das/pdxmd/body/405943427-3/0?type=med&eid=9-u1.0-_1_mt_1014924). Some doctors do not believe it exists, and I am of the opinion that it is a diagnosis indicating deeper pathology, which I find to be related to problems with mineral metabolism and mitochondrial function (Chapter 3).

Body-wide pain can manifest from various conditions, such as:

Poor Mitochondrial Function

Low Mineral Levels

Low Back Pain/Arthritis

Poor Diet

Low Vitamin D Levels

Thyroid Dysfunction

Excess Sugar in Diet

Poor Sleep (i.e. Adrenal Dysfunction, Chapter 8)

Stress

Anxiety/Depression

Inflammation

Environmental Toxin Exposures

For fibromyalgia patients, it is very important to identify the causes of pain. I generally start with making sure the patient is not eating any foods they are sensitive to, then I progress with an analysis of mitochondrial function while identifying any other sources of inflammation. I always treat the underlying conditions and this leads to the resolution or decrease in symptoms.

This condition is one of the most complicated I have ever treated, but I have found that it is treatable. The rate-limiting factor is how motivated the patient is to get better.

Treating the Cause with the Power of Belief:

Fibromyalgia is a very complex disease, but it is not impossible to treat successfully. It works best when patients are very, very motivated to get better. I have a patient who has suffered from this condition ever since she sustained a work-related injury. She has extreme pain that fluctuates in its intensity, but she never gives up from her pursuit of good health. Because she pursues, she has improved 90% since we first started working together; plus, she is identifying more and more causes of her pain. She believes, has faith, and continually puts that faith and belief into motion.

Here is what I have taught my patients to do if they suffer from Fibromyalgia:

1. Identify any possible sources of environmental toxins.

2. Avoid any and all sources of inflammation. Gluten and sugar are the most common culprits.

3. Exercise, even if it is just a short daily walk.

4. Treat any other underlying conditions, such as osteoarthritis of the spine (see Dr. Tallman for this treatment, www.arizonaprolotherapy.com).

5. Rest in between activities and take care of the liver. The liver is the energy master of the body and if its ability to metabolize environmental toxins is inhibited, pain will result.

6. Do everything possible to keep vitamin and mineral levels up. Low vitamin and mineral levels can create body-wide pain.

✌ 29 ✌
Peripheral Neuropathy

Peripheral neuropathy is defined as the dysfunction of nerves (Chapter 7), involving the axon, the nerve sheath, or both. It affects 3.5% of the population and includes symptoms such as decreased sensation, pain, tingling, burning, foot drop, or weakness (www.mdconsult.com/das/search/results/403903122-9?searchId=1412406962&k-w=peripheral%20neuropathy&area=FirstConsult&set=1&bbSearchType=single).

Peripheral Neuropathy is Diagnosed via:

EMG

Skin Sensation Testing via Physical Exam

Labs (glucose/TSH/B12/HgA1c/Sed rate/UA/genetic testing)

Nerve Conduction Studies

Diseases associated with Neuropathy include:

Diabetes

Alcoholism

Medication Side Effects

Cancer Chemotherapy

Renal Failure

Thyroid Disorders

Heavy Metal Toxicity

Cancer

Lymes Disease

HIV

Hereditary Diseases

Critical Illnesses

Guillain-Barre' Syndrome

Auto-immune Diseases

✛ Conventional Medical Treatment Options include:

Medications (i.e. Morphine, Oxycodone, Gabapentin)

✳ Alternative Medical Treatment Options include:

Acupuncture

Herbs

Supplements (i.e. Vitamins)

❂ Naturopathic Medicine, Treating the Cause:

I feel that peripheral neuropathy is actually an inflammatory disease of the mitochondria (Chapters 3 and 6). Anything that forces the body into an inflammatory state will affect those inner workings of the cells and can create ongoing inflammation. I work with patients who have peripheral neuropathy by carefully examining any causes.

Here are some I have found:

Gluten (Thurton 2013)

Low Glutathione Levels

Sugar in the Diet

Cancer Chemotherapy Medications

Medication Side Effects

Spine Disorders

Like fibromyalgia, this is very complicated to treat because it can be difficult to identify the cause. There can be an overlap in causes that create the same sensation of pain. The bottom line is that the mitochondria are not healthy, and you have to work with your Naturopathic Doctor closely to find the cause.

Treating the Cause with the Power of Belief:

This is such a difficult condition to treat much less manage the pain. I see this disease manifest after things like cancer chemotherapy or from spine disorders. But my patients believe that as I learn more about the body, I will continue to find treatments that help to lower their pain. Thus far, acupuncture, a diet free of food sensitivities and sugar, glutathione sublingual lozenges (see my website), vitamin IV infusions, and my Pitcher Plant Tincture have become some of my best friends.

Because my patients keep showing up believing I will come up with an answer for them on this very painful condition, I will continue to seek out the best treatments I can.

Here is what I have taught my patients
if they suffer from Peripheral Neuropathy:

1. Peripheral neuropathy is a disease of the mitochondria (Chapter 3).

2. Continue to nourish cells with a low inflammatory diet and lots of vitamins/minerals.

3. Keep the spine happy and in alignment with yoga.

4. Protect the feet. Wear comfortable shoes.

5. See Dr. Tallman if there are any issues of the spine that need his care (www.arizonaprolotherapy.com).

☙ 30 ❧
Multiple Sclerosis (MS)

Multiple sclerosis (MS) is defined as the demyelination and axon loss (Chapter 7) of the brain and spinal cord. It includes symptoms such as ataxia, fatigue, loss of function of joints/limbs, vision loss/changes, and vocal loss/changes. It affects 30-80/100,000 adults annually in the U.S. Most commonly MS affects those 20-40 years of age (www.mdconsult.com/das/pdxmd/body/403903122-12/1412416335?-type=med&eid=9-u1.0-_1_mt_1014469).

MS is Diagnosed via:
MRI

Lumbar Puncture for Immune/Autoimmune Cells in Central Nervous System Fluid

Conditions associated with MS include:
Other Autoimmune Diseases

Hormonal Disorders

Pain Syndromes

✛ Conventional Medical Treatment Options include:
Immune suppressive medications (i.e. Prednisone, Interferon, Glatiramer)

Counseling

Exercise

Physical Therapy

Muscle Relaxers (i.e. Baclofen)

Anti-depressants/Anti-anxiety Medications (i.e. Diazepam)

Botulinum Toxin

Anti-fatigue Medication (i.e Amantadine)

✳ Alternative Medical Treatment Options include:
Diet Changes

B12

Massage

Exercise

Supplements for Energy

✪ Naturopathic Medicine, Treating the Cause:
MS is an inflammatory disease (Horseen et al. 2012), often coming from an inability

of the patient's body to handle environmental toxins (**Pamphlett 2012 and clin**ical observation).

Patients with MS may or may not respond to an environmental detox. Some patients I have worked with had intense flares of symptoms with the application and instrumentation of simple detox tools such as use of the infrared sauna, so I am very cautious about how I proceed with them.

I have seen MS to be a disease of the liver. Patients with this condition struggle metabolizing the environmental toxins, or anything that flares their immune system. Treating the liver is very helpful in MS.

Treating the Cause with the Power of Belief:

Patient Case:

This patient started to work with me three years ago. When I first met him he had very few MS symptoms, such as a slight speech impediment and drop foot. However, the episodes of speech and gait changes started to happen more often to the point at which he went to the hospital for an IV of steroids (to stop or slow the inflammation). Initially this helped, but as time passed, he no longer responded to these types of medications (including Prednisone).

He had worked with his brother to start a granite countertop business, and I learned that in the process of both making these products and installing them, they use solvents. I worried that the MS flares started with an inability to process environmental toxins, so I started him on:

- *Infrared sauna 20 min 2-3/week followed by cold rinse in the shower.*
- *Increased antioxidants in diet (i.e. berries/greens.*
- *Supplements to help bind/eliminate toxins (i.e. Thorne Solvent Remover and Heavy Metal Detox).*
- *Dietary sugar elimination.*
- *Vitamin IV infusions (these are drips of Vitamins C/B Complex/magnesium/calcium/selenium/zinc/chromium/manganese).*

He felt great with the vitamin IV infusions but the sauna made him flare; he did not continue with the sauna, but did the IVs regularly. He also took sugar out of his diet and started juicing vegetables and berries.

The first thing I noticed was a change to his skin tone, as well as an improvement in his energy level. But, the disease continued to progress; he developed muscle spasms that began to affect his right leg. The intensity of these spasms increased over time as did the severity of his drop foot. His speech was harder to understand and honestly I was scared for him.

I could sense that if something didn't shift soon, he was headed for a wheelchair and permanent disability.

Horseen et al. (2012) explains that MS starts with inflammatory processes regulated by the immune system (Chapter 6). Once the inflammation starts, the axons of nerves are attacked (by the immune system). And once this starts, the damage to the axons essentially starves the mitochondria of the nervous system cells of sodium (Chapter 3), thereby causing more inflammation from a suffocating mitochondria: calcium levels then start to build up in the nervous system, creating an imbalance of nutrients to the mitochondria.

I decided to add an IV of normal saline to his protocol. I thought the saline (sodium) if infused into the blood directly would help support the mitochondria. It did! With just one IV of normal saline, the patient's speech improved. He said he had less saliva in the back of his throat and was able to talk clearer. I decided to infuse glutathione with the vitamin IV, thinking that since it's a detox molecule (Chapter 4) perhaps he was low. I added only a few cc's to the IV and as it got into his blood stream, the muscle spasms he was experiencing stopped. We kept up with the glutathione as an IV every 2-3 weeks.

Next, I tested the patient's testosterone levels. His testosterone was below normal, so I prescribed a testosterone gel that worked well for him to lesson fatigue. I also added my Adrenal Support Herbs, a teaspoon or two a day.

I then sent him to Dr. Tallman, DC, NMD in Scottsdale, AZ for stem cell treatments (Bonab MM. et al. 2012). Dr. Tallman uses either the patient or a donor's stem cells, and I had him introduce them to the patient's body as an epidural. We didn't see much change with the first few treatments but by the fourth there was a definite difference: the patient's balance and gait was much improved and he was re-gaining sensation to his feet.

Here is part of his story, in his words:

MS came into my life when my dad was diagnosed with it when I was sixteen. The progression of his MS was a very slow and debilitating process both mentally and physically. It took about ten years or so before it put him in a wheelchair. He has been there for the last 14 years. I've watched him go from more than capable to totally dependent on my mother for everything. I never worried that I might get it because all of dad's docs and the literature said that it was not hereditary. Imagine my surprise when I started having symptoms when I was 27. I went to my PCP and requested that I get an MRI. The results came back as consistent with MS. So I began to see a neurologist and he put me on an Interferon drug called Avonex that suppresses the immune system. I did that for about a year with no positive results. It made me feel much worse by adding flu-like symptoms and fatigue that I never thought possible. Once a week I would give myself an injection *of Interferon. As soon as the symptoms from it started to subside it was time for another shot. I saw 3 other neurologists all with the same recommendation that I get on another Interferon drug. I tried 2 more—Copaxone and Rebif. All three had the same effect on me. I gave up on them and decided to go the Naturopathic way of treatment. I found Dr. Gowey. She put me on a regimen that has been personalized for me going after the symptoms and their causes. We work on the cellular level and she pays real attention to all my questions and concerns. Attention that I never thought possible from a doctor. I was experiencing muscle spasms that my old doctor prescribed Baclofen for with little to no results. Dr. Gowey started giving me glutathione along with my multi vitamin IV's and that took away my spasms. I can actually sleep comfortably an entire night now. She also referred me to Dr. David Tallman and has been collaborating with him formulating my own stem cell treatments. I'm looking forward to the future now instead of fearing the possibilities of what might happen. I feel so blessed to have Drs Gowey and Tallman in my life. I feel much healthier now and want to let others know that there is natural relief for them, too.*

Here is what I have taught my patients to do if they struggle with MS:

1. MS is a disease of the liver that then affects the immune system, which then attacks the nervous system. Keep the liver healthy with no sugar in the diet and liver support herbs such as are found in my Immune Formula.

2. You have to do everything you can to keep inflammation low. Stay focused on a grains/dairy/sugar-free diet: no fast or processed foods.

3. Keep hormone levels healthy. I'm not sure how, but estrogen appears to help protect against MS, as women do not struggle with it as much as men do (clinical observation).

4. Stay active—physical therapy, swimming, anything you can do to keep the muscle and nervous system memory active.

5. IV nutrients are very useful, especially if low glutathione is part of the disease process (clinical observation). Low glutathione=muscle spasms in many cases (sublingual or IV is the best).

✒ 31 ✑
Insomnia

Annually, 60 million U.S. adults suffer from insomnia. Insomnia is defined as the inability to fall or stay asleep (http://www.mdconsult.com/das/pdxmd/body/403746318-3/0?type=med&eid=9-u1.0-_1_mt_1014435). Most patients with insomnia have other medical conditions that start the sleeplessness such as fibromyalgia, anxiety, depression, or pain.

Patients are Diagnosed with Insomnia via:
Sleep Study

Clinical History

In some patients insomnia starts as a child; however, for the majority of adults, onset is over the Age of 65.

✚ Conventional Medical Treatment Options include:
Medications (i.e. Trazadone, Ambien)

CPAP Machine (based on sleep study results)

✳ Alternative Medical Treatment Options include:
Herbs (i.e. Valarian, Hops)

Teas (i.e. Chamomile, Lavender)

Melatonin

Massage

Acupuncture

✿ Naturopathic Medicine, Treating the Cause:
Anything that causes a disruption in the immune (Chapter 6) or nervous systems (Chapter 7), blood sugar levels, or hormones are causes of insomnia. Adrenal cortisol elevated at night and high blood sugar are some of the most common culprits (clinical observation, Chapters 8 and 15).

Examples include:
Elevated p.m. Cortisol (Chapter 8)

Pain

Changes to Neurotransmitter Levels

Unhappiness (i.e. Depression or Anxiety)

Food Sensitivities and Processed Sugar Intake

Medications

Topical Progesterone

Testosterone Supplementation/Creams

DHEA as Supplement (it will become Cortisol)

Caffeine

Cortisol levels normally drop at night allowing you to feel drowsy. As we discussed in Chapter 8, cortisol may elevate with acute and chronic stress; however, it may also elevate from use of medications. In some women, topical progesterone may actually metabolize into elevated night cortisol. I have seen this by testing patient saliva cortisol levels after topical use. I only prescribe progesterone orally.

To Lower Elevated Night Cortisol Levels:

• Stress management (consider activities you enjoy to do, such as art, music, yoga, meditation, massage, acupuncture, or counseling).

• Bio or neurofeedback.

• Integrative Therapeutics Cortisol Manager (helps re-sensitize hypothalamus receptors to the presence of elevated cortisol); I prescribe this to patients for use before bedtime.

• Adrenal support herbs used in the morning only, when cortisol is naturally supposed to be higher.

• Switch to oral progesterone as opposed to topical.

• Pain management.

Pain, as from arthritis, fibromyalgia, or peripheral neuropathy, keeps patients up at night. You can try pain management via medications or medical marijuana, but I usually send patients to see Dr. David Tallman, DC, NMD (www.arizonaprolotherapy.com) for prolotherapy. He treats causes of the joint pains by restoring the body's infrastructure (i.e. spine) back to normal alignment.

Elevated neurotransmitters (Chapter 7) may also keep you up at night. Norepinephrine or epinephrine are both released by the adrenals in response to acute stressors, and can make you feel "amped". GABA is a neurotransmitter that can make you feel relaxed; if it is too low you may feel anxious.

To Balance Neurotransmitter Levels:

• Test neurotransmitter levels via urine testing. With these results, your Naturopathic physician can then use amino acid or vitamin/mineral therapies to balance your neurotransmitters.

• Increase mineral levels (minerals such as magnesium are needed to build neurotransmitters).

• Increase vitamin levels (vitamins such as the B's and Vitamin C are needed to build neurotransmitters).

• If GABA is low, medications such as Ambien may help, although they may become addicting, so I do not generally advise their use. You can also purchase GABA in health food stores as a supplement. Medical marijuana is a plant that helps to increase GABA levels (Grotenhermen and Russo 2002).

• Bio and Neurofeedback therapies may help you shift neurotransmitter levels. As a medical student I did a rotation at an Integrative Department at a hospital in Minneapolis, MN. The therapists used biofeedback techniques to teach children how to be in control of their emotions/reactions to stress; their results were impressive.

Balancing our neurotransmitters is important, but don't ignore your spiritual or emotional side. In Eastern Medical terms, each organ in your body has a very special purpose (energetically) beyond its physiological function. The liver is one of the biggest movers of energy, and is spiritually responsible for helping you manifest the purpose for your life. Acupuncture came out of the Taoist philosophy that says we all come with a purpose (Chapter 9). If you are not listening to your path or not following it, you will not sleep well—you will toss and turn or not fall to sleep easily. Not following your path disrupts your heart (the energy around your heart, your "Shen" in Chinese medicine).

To address this, I use the following:
Acupuncture
Chinese Herbal Blends
Counseling
Spiritual Counseling/Guidance
Retreats
My Immune Formula (has a lot of liver support herbs in it)

Food sensitivities can keep you up at night because they are causing an inflammatory reaction. A common one is sugar.

The best treatments are:
Avoiding Foods you are sensitive to
Avoiding Sugar (Processed Sugar)
Avoid Alcohol (too sugary, will wake you up at night)

If you want to use herbs to help you relax before you go to sleep, remember it is not truly Naturopathic unless the herbs are treating one of the causes just discussed (or another cause). I generally use herbs after I am working with the patient on the cause. Oftentimes, I use herbs to lower night blood sugars or inflammation. I find that high sugars and inflammation are the main causes of insomnia. Or, cortisol is too high at night. Integrative Therapeutics makes a product called "Cortisol Manager" which is good at helping lower night cortisol. It oftentimes takes several months of use of this product before a difference is noted, but some patients respond upon the first dose.

Treating the Cause with the Power of Belief:

A lot of people feel really hopeless about insomnia. They feel they will never have a good night's sleep. Not my patients. They believe, so they keep showing up until we figure out why they are not sleeping.

I can think of two patients in particular who staunchly believed they would sleep a perfect night, and soon! They were right. I had put them both on liver supportive therapies (castor oil packs in one case, and my Immune Formula in another case) and BOTH patients started to sleep through the night via treatment of the liver! This made me think back to my acupuncture training: the liver is a powerful energy mover, and especially at night (if it is not in balance).

Here is what I have taught my patients to do
if they suffer from Insomnia:

1. Support the liver! My Immune Formula is awesome for this purpose.

2. Use castor oil packs before bed (Chapter 35).

3. Avoid consumption of processed sugars and alcohol before bed. Sugar will keep you up at night (clinical observation).

4. Treat your adrenals well. Read my mom's book on the adrenals, *Zip and Zap Take a Nap*, available in bookstores everywhere.

5. Keep your heart happy. Follow your purpose!

6. Exercise—a lot! Balanced exercise will help you sleep like a baby!

❧ 32 ❧
Bipolar

Bipolar is characterized and defined as mania (euphoria) alternating with episodes of depression (loss of pleasure in life or suicidality). 800 (per 100,000) in the U.S. annually have bipolar syndrome, and 100 a year (of 100,000) are diagnosed. Causes are considered "unknown" (www.mdconsult.com/das/pdxmd/body/405410255-5/1418023963?-type=med&eid=9-u1.0-_1_mt_1014421).

Bipolar is Diagnosed via:
Clinical History/Review of Symptoms
CBC/CMP/Thyroid Panel/Liver Panel in Blood Work
Drug Testing

✚ Conventional Medical Treatment Options include:
Lithium
Counseling
Anti-depressant Medications (i.e. Wellbutrin)

✳ Alternative Medical Treatment Options include:
Reiki
Massage
Acupuncture
Herbs

☻ Naturopathic Medicine, Treating the Cause:
I think bipolar comes from problems with hormone metabolism (Chapter 8) and processed sugar in the diet. I always check hormone levels when helping patients diagnosed with bipolar syndrome. More often than not I find elevated testosterone (in women); or, I find that hormones fluctuate (doesn't this sound like PMS, perimenopause or andropause?).

I also see that people who are bipolar tend to eat poorly (i.e. too many simple carbs such as processed sugars and wheat products). They are very sensitive to the slightest changes in diet and shifting hormone levels.

In working with patients who have been diagnosed as Bipolar I:
- Run levels of testosterone/estrogen/progesterone via blood.
- Consider treatment of thyroid/adrenals.

- Test cortisol via saliva test.

- Eliminate processed sugar from diet.

- Treat liver with my Immune Formula, a combo of liver/immune support.

Treating the Cause with the Power of Belief:

Patient Testimonial:

I am 54 years old and have suffered from depression for over 20 years. I was put on many drugs, but none helped. As time passed I was diagnosed as being bipolar.

My counselor suggested I see Dr. Gowey, which I felt was a last resort. I had been to see so many other professionals, doctors, and counselors, that I was starting to feel "what for, how can she help", not even thinking about my three beautiful children and grandchildren. I was at a point where I was thinking that my life was over and that my dog even needed to find a new home. I was on so many medications I couldn't even remember all the names, but none helped and only made me feel worse. I felt like the living dead. My economic situation had gotten worse, too, with all my health struggles. I had started and stopped many businesses but lost money on all of them and decided to go on disability in 2003.

Dr. Gowey began to work with me and put me on things like B vitamins and herbs. She also encouraged me to change my diet to foods that were less inflammatory. After working with me for a bit she added acupuncture to my protocol, and that was a really incredible experience. At the first session, I could feel some sort of energy on special points like something was being released from my body. That sensation of well-being lasted all week. I started to feel different, started to go walking, got out of the house more; I could see sunshine coming into my life instead of so many dark clouds.

I had checked hormone levels in this patient and her pituitary hormones were elevated. This is most likely what was causing symptoms. Currently, I am sending her for an MRI and other relevant testing to rule out cancer. But the point remains: bipolar may have a cause. Work with your Naturopathic Doctor to find it.

Here is what I have taught my patients to do if they suffer from Bipolar Disorder:

1. Keep vitamin/mineral levels high.

2. Keep processed sugar out of the diet.

3. Keep hormone levels healthy. Nourish the adrenal glands.

4. Exercise.

5. Find a community you feel you belong to. Invest in your community.

6. Find someone in your life you trust to help you monitor your symptoms, and have them help you watch for major swings in your mood. This will help you identify causes.

❧ 33 ❧
Behavioral Problems in Children

"Behavioral" problems in children is a classification involving several conditions such as autism, ADD, ADHD, or depression.

Behavioral Issues are Diagnosed via:
Physician or Therapist Behavioral Evaluation

✚ Conventional Medical Treatment Options include:
Medications (i.e. Ritalin)

Counseling

Behavioral Modification Therapy

✳ Alternative Medical Treatment Options include:
Herbs

Supplements (i.e. Vitamins)

✿ Naturopathic Medicine, Treating the Cause:
Children act out because something in their system is out of balance. This can come from different sources and can be very difficult to identify. Here are some possibilities that I have seen clinically:

• Children need lots of nutritional support. Processed sugars cause behavioral problems/anxiety/depression/hyperactivity/diabetes.

• Vaccines are a problem only if the child has abnormal detox pathways (i.e. mitochondrial function is low/abnormal, Chapter 3).

• Children need lots of emotional support.

• Children need adrenal support. Kids are overworked (too much school activities, not enough rest) so the adrenals burn out early in life. I put kids on my adrenal herbs with great outcomes. My mom and I wrote a children's book on adrenal fatigue. I recommend you read it over with your kids (*Zip and Zap Take a Nap*). It is available in bookstores everywhere.

I think most of these conditions come from problems with the adrenals (Chapter 8).

❧ Happy Adrenals = Happy Life ❧

Treating the Cause with the Power of Belief:

Patient Case:

One of my patients brought in her six-year-old daughter for treatment of temper tantrums. This child had a tendency to scream, yell, beat on doors or walls, and challenge her mom when she didn't get her way. She also tended to be very tired, sleeping up to 11 hours a night. She challenged her mom (my patient) a lot but didn't challenge her dad. Initially, I put the child on the homeopathic remedy called Carcinosin, indicated when someone needs to feel in control of their situation. The child responded favorably to the remedy but she still was having outbursts, although not as dramatic.

I kept the child on the remedy for a few months and then decided to add herbs and vitamins. For some reason, I thought to add my adrenal herbs mostly because the child would have outbursts if she felt out-of-control (which can arise from hormonal imbalances in the adrenals, Chapter 8).

Mom notified me that within a short period of time her child was much calmer; three months later she called me to report that her daughter was "like a new child." She was no longer having outbursts and was very respectful of her mom. The mom reported they were no longer having "issues" as long as she stayed on the herbs!

Here is what I have taught my patients to do if they struggle with Behavioral Issues in their Children:

1. Don't forget to consider adrenal support if you have a child that is acting out of turn or has outbursts. Look deeper with these conditions and find a good Naturopathic Physician to work with.

2. Try Social Thinking. See Chapter 34 for details.

Please read the following from Dr. Mike Knapp, NMD

The terms ADD (Attention Deficit Disorder) and ADHD (Attention Deficit Hyperactivity Disorder) are often used interchangeably. ADD specifically refers to inattentive behavior with a lack of hyperactivity whereas ADHD has this as a major feature along with inattention. There is great overlap in the symptoms and they are often difficult to completely differentiate, as these are largely different aspects of the same problem. For simplicity, both states will be referred to as ADHD.

Classic symptoms of ADHD include an inability to focus and complete tasks in a timely manner, difficulty with organization, easy distraction, poor listening, and forgetfulness in daily activities (American Psychiatric Association 2000). The hyperactivity component is usually characterized by restlessness with the inability to sit for any period of time, constant motion of the hands, feet, or body, and excessive talking.

ADHD has been thought of as a childhood disorder but more recent evidence suggests that symptoms persist in adulthood for about 50% of people (Wodushek and Neumann 2003). Adults are commonly treated with anti-depressant drugs and/or similar stimulant medications that are used for children. Symptoms of ADHD may be more difficult to recognize in adults because they develop and adapt behaviors that are deemed more acceptable based on cultural norms. Hyperactivity can then appear as symptoms of generalized anxiety and restlessness. The chronic nature of ADHD means that many people may continue to suffer in adulthood with decreased work performance and inability to keep track of bills and financial responsibilities.

Many people with ADHD also suffer from other disorders (Krull 2014). Oppositional Defiant Disorder (ODD) and Conduct Disorder are separate but overlapping conditions that show persistent and unacceptable behaviors with regard to defying authority. In addition, Conduct Disorder displays a violation of rules that escalates to bullying, cruelty, and property destruction. Other conditions that frequently appear with ADHD include anxiety, depression, antisocial personality disorder, and learning disabilities such as dyslexia.

Genetics appear to play a role in the development of ADHD (Krull 2014). Currently, we can't change our genes (and I would be very hesitant to undergo such treatment!), but family history gives us information about a child's potential susceptibilities. Also, Naturopathic Doctors understand that we can change the way our genes are expressed. This is a fascinating field of research termed "epigenetics" and it is proof that what you do makes a difference. Our environment, physical activity, and the food we eat on a daily basis all affect the way our genes are expressed, which then affects our state of health or disease. There are other risk factors beyond genetics. Both alcohol and tobacco exposure during pregnancy have shown increased risk for children to develop ADHD (Substance Abuse and Mental Health Services Administration 2011). Alcohol is associated with a range of health problems termed Fetal Alcohol Spectrum Disorder, which may include physical deformities and abnormal brain development leading to mental impairments. Other drugs, particularly methamphetamine, are known neurotoxins that can affect the structure and function of the brain in the developing fetus (Jansson 2014). According to the 2010 National Survey on Drug Use and Health, substance use of women age 15-44 years old during pregnancy was as follows: 16.3% cigarettes, 10.8% alcohol, and 4.4% illicit drugs (Substance Abuse and Mental Health Services Administration 2011). These numbers indicate that a substantial minority of children are born each year with risk of neurological disorders and ADHD that may have been preventable. Lead exposure during childhood has also been linked with ADHD. Children are at greater risk for lead toxicity because they absorb significantly more lead through the intestines than adults.

Medications

Conventional Medical treatment usually consists of stimulant drugs (Ritalin), non-stimulant drugs (Strattera), or anti-depressive drugs (Bupropion) targeting neurotransmitters that alter our brain chemistry to help control impulses and increase attention. Some patients experience great benefit from these medications, but other effects of drug therapy must also be considered. Anti-depressant drugs cannot be stopped abruptly and require the supervision of a doctor to safely stop or change to a different therapy. Therefore, this tends to be a long-term treatment and patient compliance is important. There has been debate over whether Ritalin treatment increases the risk of future alcohol and substance abuse disorders. At worst, patients could be trading one mental health condition for another. A less controversial topic is the abuse of Ritalin by patients dispersing their prescriptions to others for recreational use or for use as a study-aid (Wilens et al. 2008). Research at a German university showed that in the previous year, 20% of students had used someone else's prescription drug to help them study. This doesn't take into account those using stimulants to "get high". Also, misuse of stimulant drugs greatly increases the risk of adverse effects. Adverse reactions to ADHD medications include liver damage, high blood pressure, irregular heart rhythms, stunted growth, and suicidal ideation. Though prescribing practices have not changed since the FDA announced these recent warnings, the risks and benefits should be weighed based on individual needs, and non-drug treatments should be given consideration.

Importance of a Holistic Treatment Plan

Some of the symptoms of ADHD are normal for kids just being kids, but for those with true ADHD this leads to poor performance in school, hindered social development, and can add significant stress to the household. Drugs are rarely the complete answer to chronic health issues. Naturopathic care bridges multiple disciplines to provide gentle, effective long-term support as part of an individualized approach to the management of ADHD and accompanying disorders.

Counseling or therapy is important to modify the home environment, help children learn to take responsibility for choices, and work with low self-esteem that often accompanies ADHD (Krull 2014). Behavior modifications can add structure to the child's routine and give parents new tools in responding to behaviors so that new positive outcomes are possible. In some cases, the creation of an individual educational plan (IEP) through the school can provide added resources tailored to the specific areas the child is struggling within the educational process.

Diet modification and the identification of nutritional deficiencies can be very beneficial in managing symptoms (Hoffer 2005). Food intolerances (sensitivities) are non-allergy reactions to food in the body, which cause symptoms that range from belching and bloating, to migraine headaches, mood, and behavior changes. Foods commonly associated with ADHD are food additives, preservatives and dyes, sugars, and milk or dairy products. Further, tartrazine (yellow dye #5) is a common food dye that was shown to have a strong affect on the brain of mice. It impaired memory, learning responses, and increased inflammation was observed in brain tissue (Gao et al. 2011). Tartrazine also decreases function of the body's protective antioxidant systems that may lead to mild ongoing damage to brain cells (Abd and Moram et al. 2012). Food intolerances and additives are not the cause of ADHD but elimination of offending foods from the diet can significantly decrease symptoms.

Nutritional supplements can also play a role in managing ADHD. Careful and individualized selection is important to minimize costs, and because compliance with multiple supplements is difficult for many children. Essential fatty acids, zinc, or amino acids have been shown effective in placebo-controlled trials and have minimal side effects (Milte et al. 2012; Huss et al. 2010; Krull 2014; Hoffer 2005). Fish oil (an essential fatty acid) promotes healthy nerves and can be beneficial when inflammation is contributing to symptoms. Zinc is a very common nutrient deficiency because of the poor nutrient content in the soil of most large-scale farms.

Constitutional homeopathy is a cost-effective tool that can be very effective for managing the symptoms of ADHD and treating the underlying imbalances that may be present in these children (Pellow et al. 2011). We can gently achieve remarkable changes in behavior without aggressively manipulating brain chemistry in the way drugs intend. Compliance is also quite good because the medicines are well tolerated and have no offensive taste.

Case Study

The following is a case example from my clinic. While there are cases that respond with extraordinary success in a strikingly short time, this case is intended to illustrate the outcomes we can routinely come to achieve through Naturopathic care.

Initial Consultation – 8/2012

A colleague referred "H" to me for constitutional homeopathic care. Her main complaint at this time was ADHD and she was also under Naturopathic treatment for hypothyroidism. She was fidgety with difficulty paying attention in school and in her online classes. She was unable to take tests unless they were administered in a quiet room away from other students. She also had impulsiveness in her speech. Words would come out of her mouth before she could think about the consequences to herself and others, which she would then quickly regret. She had previously been prescribed the medication Straterra which was helpful for her symptoms, but she soon developed high blood pressure and tachycardia (fast heart rate) from it, so her parents were seeking a different mode of treatment.

One of the most problematic symptoms for the family were daily episodes of sudden anger and fear with yelling and hitting, which she would not remember.

Little is known if H's family history beyond her mother's substance abuse issues and that she was exposed to alcohol, methamphetamine, and other drugs throughout the pregnancy. She was adopted at 6 weeks old. The effects of various drug exposures during development on mood, attention/cognition, and physical health are difficult to separate from potentially inherited risk for ADHD and other mental disorders. Her doctors did believe that her severe life-long constipation was due to nerve damage in the colon from drug exposure.

I prescribed homeopathic Stramonium 200c in 1oz of water (10 drops 3 times weekly).

Follow-up #1 - 9/2012

H experienced a rapid decrease in frequency of the anger episodes and her previous inability to remember what she had said and done had completely resolved. She was able to be calmer, less impulsive with thoughts and speech, and was able to communicate better with her family. She was still having much difficulty with focusing on school and other short tasks, but her memory had improved.

H's treatment hit a roadblock immediately after the death of her counselor and close family friend. She quickly developed walking pneumonia, became very sad and withdrawn, and wanted to spend most of her time alone in her room. School was very difficult and she felt she had to "wear a mask" all day to keep up her appearances and avoid unwanted attention from classmates. Hiding her feelings all day was exhausting and she would come home and blow up at her family.

Stramonium was not helping with the acute stress of the death of her friend, so I changed the prescription to homeopathic Ignatia 200c in 1oz of water taken 10 drops daily. The pneumonia was treated at an urgent care clinic previous to this visit.

Follow-up #2 – 10/2012

H's mood improved within 2 days of starting the Ignatia. She was much happier, wanted to engage with friends again and school was less stressful. Her attention was also improved and although she still felt a restless sensation in her feet, she was able to concentrate and do her work. Grades that were previously Ds and Fs were raised to Cs.

The Ignatia was continued because she was showing steady improvement.

Follow-up #3 – 1/2013

H had maintained improvement for several months with her symptoms of restlessness and inattention. She was able to pass the driver's test to get her license, which was previously a source of much anxiety. H had decided to leave her high school because of their repeated inability to comply with the individualized education plan (IEP) that her parents and the school had agreed upon. She was registered to take the GED exam (given over 3 days) and had applied for special testing accommodations so that she could be given the test in a quiet room. Test taking had been significantly more difficult since she had been the victim of sexual abuse the previous year. In most situations, she felt anxious and unable to concentrate because of recurrent thoughts that people around her might hurt her. Anger, road rage, and changeable mood, had begun to be a frequent problem again. Episodes were not as intense as previously, and she was able to remember her actions, but, they were troubling to family life. In addition to homeopathic treatment, I began overseeing all of H's chronic health complaints and we decided to investigate food intolerances that could be contributing to her mood, weight gain, and poor digestion.

It appeared that H had gotten good benefit from the Ignatia for several months, but a new medicine was needed to keep her progress moving, so I prescribed homeopathic Kali bromatum, to be taken similar to the previous medicines. Re-establishing a relationship with a counselor was also emphasized to further address anger, anxiety, and her history of abuse.

Follow-up #4 – 2/2013

H was able to concentrate and did well on her GED exam despite being denied private testing accommodations. School and study is still not easy, but she is able to apply herself and achieve outcomes that were very difficult in the past. She has the confidence to begin attending beauty school as training for her future profession.

The results of the food intolerance panel came back showing marked reactions to soy, wheat, eggs, and all milk products. Due to the identification of multiple food sensitivities we began treatment for leaky gut syndrome as follows:

1. Strict removal of all offending foods, food colorings, and preservatives for eight weeks.

2. Probiotics daily for improving gut bacteria.

3. HCl and digestive enzyme supplement before each meal to aid in breaking down food and increase absorption of nutrients in a weak digestive tract.

4. Intestinal repair powder 2-3 times daily to repair the damage of the intestinal lining caused by chronic food intolerances.

Conclusion

H recognized correlations in the stability of her mood with maintaining avoidance of her food triggers and sudden aggravations in mood and behavior after consuming them. With avoidance of these foods, she lost 20 lbs that were contributing to frequent back pain and fatigue. This weight loss will also decrease her risk of diabetes and other future illness.

H's ADHD is currently well controlled. She has a complicated health history and continues to need ongoing treatment, but her success illustrates the necessity of developing and adapting a long-term plan. Long-standing health complaints are often far more deep reaching than a single main symptom and cure is not something achieved overnight.

Find Dr. Knapp, NMD at Root Natural Health, www.rootnaturalhealth.com.

Part III

Treat the Person, Not the Disease

In this section, I discuss ways Naturopathic Medicine can be used to stimulate the body to heal itself. I grouped treatments under categories. The categories pertain to building, nourishing, and shifting patient energy or constitution so that they may move out of their "disease", or maintain health despite their "disease." I combine treatments depending on what patients need.

I also do not see patients as diseases. I see them as people with need of nourishment, shifting, or building.

✎ 34 ✎
Building Treatments

1. Glutathione

Glutathione is a detox molecule (Chapter 4) located in every cell of your body. It is highly concentrated in your liver, lungs, and gut. It is composed primarily of three amino acids and Vitamin C. Its job is to bind to toxins in order to help your body eliminate things like environmental pollutants. Patients often tell me they want to "detox" their liver. I encourage them to think of "building the liver" and detoxing the body.

In Chapter 4, I discussed how I have prescribed glutathione for patients and the mixed results I get. If you use this molecule as part of your treatment regime, I recommend you first consult with a Naturopathic Physician familiar with detox pathways. Have them take a thorough medical history before glutathione is prescribed.

2. Botanical Medicine

Herbs are building and nourishing. Used in the right way, they can create subtle, positive changes. Herbs can be used to treat symptoms, but I prefer to use them to build the body and strengthen energy. I don't prescribe herbs in a tablet or powdered form (unless the powder is for tea, as in slippery elm). Liquid herbs (tinctures) absorb the best.

Here are some of my Favorite Herbs:
- **Avena**—for calming and building the adrenal glands
- **Ginseng**—for energizing and building the adrenal glands
- **Ashwaghanda**—for strengthening and building the adrenal glands
- **Rhodiola**—for encouraging endurance and building the adrenal glands
- **Licorice**—for building the adrenal glands
- **Lemon Balm**—for building the nervous system
- **Ginger**—for building the immune system
- **Ginkgo**—for building the circulatory system
- **Dandelion**—for building the liver
- **Milk Thistle**—for building the liver
- **Astragalus**—for building the immune system
- **Echinacea Root**—for building the immune system

- **Goldenseal**—for building the immune system
- **Pitcher Plant**—for building the inner workings of the cell (Harris et al. 2012)

Herbs like friends. They don't like to work alone; I rarely prescribe just one. You can view my formulas at www.goweyresearchgroup.com.

3. Vitamin IV Infusions (Meyer's Cocktail)

These are awesome! Build the body by getting vitamins and minerals to the tissues—that is my mantra. So many suffer from gut disorders, which means vitamin and mineral absorption will be low. Low vitamins and minerals=chronic diseases. I prescribe vitamin IVs for patients with chronic fatigue (GREAT for this) and conditions whereby absorption of nutrients is low such as in IBS.

Here are Nutrients that can be added to a Vitamin IV:

Vitamin C	Magnesium	Zinc
B Complex	Calcium	Trace Minerals
Extra B12	Selenium	(such as Manganese)

4. Building Foods

Eating well is the most important thing you can do for your body next to exercising and keeping a positive mind-set.

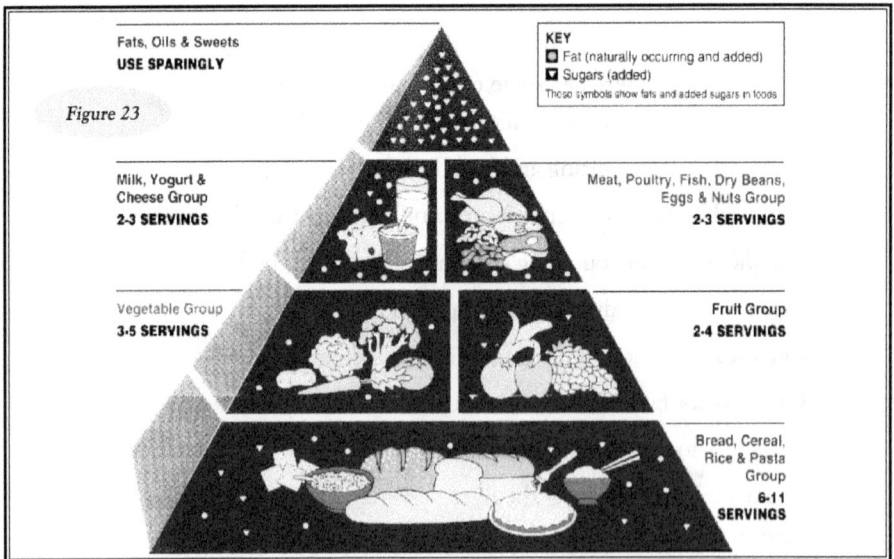

Figure 23. This is the USDA's 1992 version of the right foods to eat (www.en.wikipedia.org/wiki/File:USDA_Food_Pyramid.

This food pyramid focuses on refined carbohydrates as the most important food group to eat daily at 6-11 servings, followed by some fruit, some veggies, a lot of protein (meats, dairy), and some fats.

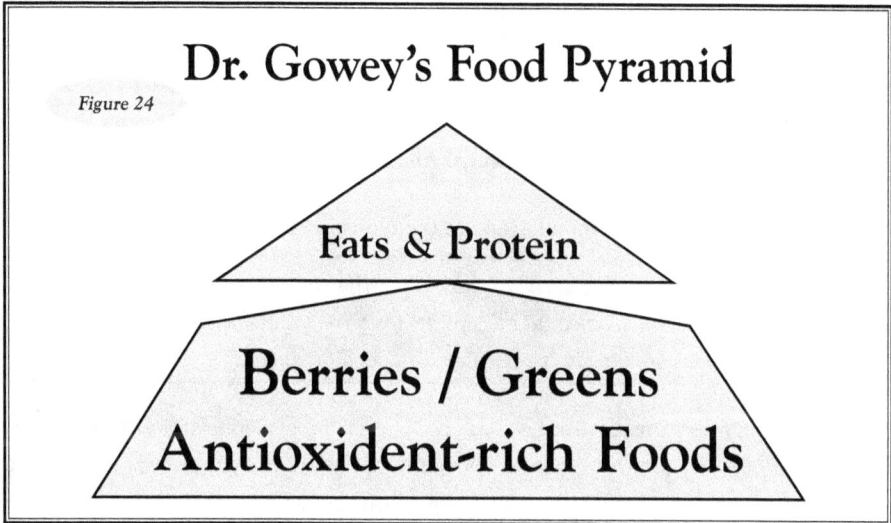

Dr. Gowey's Food Pyramid

Figure 24

Fats & Protein

Berries / Greens
Antioxident-rich Foods

☞ *In contrast, Figure 24 shows Dr. Gowey's Food Pyramid*

I put antioxidant-rich foods such as berries and greens on the bottom and at the highest percentage of the diet because they are the most important to our bodies. Fats come next and protein-rich foods come last. Fats and protein need to be balanced relative to each other; meaning you can eat similar percents of each relative to your total caloric intake. The antioxidant foods are definitely the most important. You need antioxidants to induce apoptosis (Chapter 5). I don't put grains of any kind on this Pyramid. It is not because I don't eat them occasionally, it is because people eat too many grains and they are not necessary. Some rice or quinoa as an occasional additive to a meal I think is fine, but don't make these foods one of your main food groups. They tend to promote inflammation (personal and clinical experience). I also don't put dairy on this Pyramid. Dairy can create a lot of adverse symptoms such as sinus infections, ear infections, constipation, and asthma (especially in children).

There is research behind dairy and high protein contributing to cancer (Campbell and Campbell 2006; Kroenke et al. 2013). You need antioxidants (Chapter 5) in vegetables and fruits to lower inflammation, prevent cancer, and maintain normal cell function. Antioxidant-rich foods promote a process called "apoptosis". Apoptosis is the process that signals cell death (in a damaged cell). This is something that happens only with the color rich pigments in foods like berries. If your antioxidant load is low, then the probability of a cell to stay abnormal is very high; this is part of the start of cancer and any kind of chronic disease.

I think the right dietary fats are extremely important. Omega oils (Chapter 1) build cell membranes which means they help with neurotransmitter function, hormone function, memory, mood, and immune system regulation. Too many people eat oils that have been heated and then packaged. I did an experiment once where I avoided chips (we all love our chips, don't we) for a few months and then had a bag of corn chips. Tasted great but I gained a few pounds and noticed a change to my skin. My assistant Dianna notices a reduction in her memory when she eats potato chips.

My recommendation: Make chips on your own.

You can do this by cutting corn tortillas into strips and then pan-frying for a few minutes at a low heat with coconut oil. A very tasty treat and does not seem to create the inflammation as do already fried-and-packed food products do.

Processed sugars are really hard on the body, even processed grains. I tell patients it is wisest not to eat anything out of a box, and to really limit the sweet treats. If you start to scrutinize labels you will see just how many foods have added sugar.

I have seen that sugar (even low antioxidant fruits in the diet) contribute to more than just diabetes. Patients with varying medical concerns all had elevated or elevating levels of HgA1c. HgA1c is a red blood cell coated in sugars. I think when our bodies have to process sugar too often, the body starts to stick them on red blood cells not knowing where else to put them. This, I theorize, starts an inflammatory response.

Protein is a necessary building block of the body (such as in cell membranes, Chapter 1) but it also builds the immune system (Chapter 6). Inflammatory cells are made from protein, as are cell signalers. Too much protein could push the inflammatory pathways. I recommend patients watch their protein intake. It may be wise to occasionally protein fast if they are dealing with a chronic disease like cancer or obesity. "Weight is Inflammation", I tell all my patients. It is inflammation pushed by protein (and the wrong fats). Drop your protein and that will help tremendously.

5. Mind/Body Mind-set

When patients speak negatively about themselves, I can feel that like a ton of bricks hitting me. It is awful. Negativity limits my ability to find research that will help. If you want to be well, you have to have the vision of what that looks like in your mind; otherwise no one, not even your physician, can help you.

Please do yourself and those around you a favor: shift.

Start by shifting the subconscious messages by using imagery and pictures to change.

Stare at those pictures or images, put them in picture frames, and look at them daily. Meditate on them. Over time you will realize your attitude is changing for the better. Do the same with money and finances (Osteen 2013). If you believe you don't have money, you won't. Money is just energy and you have to let it flow. Have gratitude even for small things. It is the small things that make life so good. For me, it's a little cup of green tea here and there throughout my day that makes things so nice.

6. Build Your Community by Thinking Socially

We all need to give and receive love. Love builds! Having a strong sense of community in your life will help you feel great. Social Thinking helps create this community.

My friend Laura Brummels is an advocate of "Social Thinking". She is a Speech Pathologist who has spent her career teaching patients with ADD, ADHD, and Spectrum Disorders how to move successfully through life by thinking through the eyes of others. She finds that those with Spectrum Disorders do better if they can get out of thinking just about themselves.

Laura Brummels' Thoughts on Social Thinking

Social Thinking is what we do when we interact with people: we think about them. And how we think about people affects how we behave, which in turn affects how others respond to us, which in turn affects our own emotions. Whether we are with friends, sending an email, in a classroom, or at the grocery store, we take in the thoughts, emotions, and intentions of the people we are interacting with. Most of us have developed our communications sense from birth onwards, steadily observing and acquiring social information and learning how to respond to people. Because social thinking is an intuitive process, we usually take it for granted.

This often has nothing to do with conventional measures of intelligence. In fact, many people score high on IQ and standardized tests, yet do not intuitively learn the nuances of social communication and interactions. How do we develop a treatment for those who have social learning challenges? To explain this, we use the analogy of a tree that develops a strong root system and trunk before it can grow healthy branches and leaves. Progressive social thinking and related social skills grow out of a strong root system and solid trunk, from which sturdy branches develop that produce healthy leaves. This process is called "teaching at the roots".

For example, several of my students with a history of "social skills" training will enter the treatment room, greet me, and never make eye contact. It wasn't until the concept "eyes have thoughts" was introduced that they began to understand that the reason we make eye contact is because eye gaze is a likely indicator of what people are thinking about. And when we are having a conversation, listening to the teacher, playing a game, etc., it is expected that we think about them. But since we can't see thoughts, we have to show them with our eyes.

Social Thinking is a very unique treatment program; it helps clients better understand why thinking from the eyes of others is important, which will in turn, make it easier on the individual as they navigate the world we live in.

For more information, visit www.socialthinking.com.

❧ 35 ❧
Treatments that Nourish

1. Castor Oil Packs

Promoted by Edgar Cayce (www.edgarcayce.org/are/holistic_health/data/thcast1. html), castor oil soaks well into the skin when applied topically with heat. Castor oil is termed a "lymphagogue", meaning it stimulates the movement and workings of lymphocytes, the types of immune cells that sit in tissues until they are needed (Chapter 6) to fight infections. The lymphocytes remind me of Pac Man ghosts that sit and wait in the little box on the screen until they launch to go after the Mr. or Ms. Pac Mans. Castor oil gets these "ghosts" moving into the circulation to do their job of reducing inflammation, responding to bacteria/viruses, or helping repair tissues.

Cayce tells people on his website to do the packs with a heating pad, but I don't feel it wise to use electricity over the liver.

I recommend the following:

Castor Oil Pack

1. *Apply castor oil to skin over liver, tissue, or joint you are wanting to treat.*
2. *Cover area with a thin cloth.*
3. *Cover with a hot water bottle.*
4. *Rest 10-15 minutes.*
5. *Repeat daily or as needed.*

Some of my patients tell me this helps them fall to sleep at night, while others use it to stimulate a stubborn menstrual cycle or reduce effects of PMS/perimenopause. No matter how you decide to use it, never use castor oil for active infections, as it will cause them to spread. If you need, I have a talk on Blog Talk Radio on how to do a castor oil pack. Follow me as "NIdoc" on Blog Talk to listen and learn!

I developed a pitcher plant-infused castor oil that is even more effective than castor oil alone. I prescribe it for joint pains and have seen it dramatically reduce anything from osteoarthritic related pain to menstrual cramps. You can find it at www.goweyresearchgroup.com.

2. Home Hydrotherapy

Your immune system can be supported by use of a simple tool: water.

Principles applicable in water therapies are:

- Heat dilates vessels, bringing circulation to the area.

- Cold initially constricts vessels, then dilates to warm the area (this is a pumping action that also brings circulation to the area).

- Alternating hot and cold brings the most circulation to the area because of the heat (dilating) and cold (constricting then dilating) causing movement of blood.

- Circulating blood brings white blood cells that can boost the immune system.

General rules of thumb for hydrotherapy applications are:

- Never put wet cotton on dry cotton (can make your skin feel clammy).

- Never use water that is scalding hot.

- Never use towels that are too cold (not so cold they are crunchy).

- If the cold towel or application does not warm after 10 minutes, keep on for another 10 minutes. A non-warming cold application means your energy is too low to warm the towel. Leaving the cold on longer will help boost your immune system more.

- Enjoy the process.

Wet Socks
This treatment moves circulation and lymph cells, great for sinus infections.
1. *Get a pair of cotton socks.*
2. *Get them nice and cold and wet (but not so cold they crinkle).*
3. *Put on your feet.*
4. *Cover with wool socks.*
5. *Rest 20 minutes.*

Warming Compress
This treatment brings circulation to the throat, great for sore throats.
1. *Get a cold washcloth (wet, not sopping wet).*
2. *Place on throat.*
3. *Cover with wool or fleece.*
4. *Rest 20 minutes.*
5. *May repeat often.*

Warming T-shirt

This treatment is for coughs, fevers, and colds.

1. *Get a cotton t-shirt.*

2. *Get this shirt cold and wet.*

3. *Wring out well.*

4. *Put on.*

5. *Cover with wool or fleece.*

6. *Rest 20 minutes or go to sleep with it on (Boyle and Saine 1988; Kneipp 1980; Davidson 1960).*

Here are a few treatments I like to prescribe for patients:

3. Keep Inflammation Low

The easiest way to lower systemic inflammation is to do your best to avoid foods your body may be sensitive to. There are many different types of food sensitivities. The most common are called delayed sensitivity reactions and involve a cell in your immune system called an IgG. There are four of these. When you eat a food you are sensitive to, your immune cells (the IgGs) will react by binding to the food. This is the start of the inflammatory process that takes different lengths of time depending on the type of IgG that reacts. IgG 1 reactions occur relatively quickly (within an hour) whereas an IgG 4 will take a few days to occur. This means you may have symptoms within an hour to a few days.

There are a few specialty labs that can test for IgG levels, such as US Biotek or Immunolabs. I use Immunolabs. Skin testing does NOT identify these IgG 1-4 reactions.

4. Maintain Homeostasis

I use saline IVs for patients who have inflammatory disorders such as MS, fatty liver, HTN, or kidney diseases. This sounds simple, but if you nourish the inner workings of the cell with an isotonic solution, it is easier to implement other treatments.

5. Balance and Nourish the Yin and Yang Energies *(Chi)*

As a practitioner of acupuncture, I am continually amazed by how well this modality helps my patients. How does it work? I am always asked that question and I wish there was a concrete way to answer. Acupuncture restores the normal flow of energy through our bodies that lifestyle, overwork, injuries, or stress either changes or diminishes.

Our bodies have highway-like systems of energy flowing from our skin to various organs. Needles restore the flow of that energy when properly placed in the skin by a licensed provider. Massage, meditation, and yoga work on similar energetic platforms to help nourish our energy. "Dry needling" done by physical therapists I never, ever prescribe or endorse. These providers have not had the extensive training necessary for the proper application of needles.

You have two primary forms of energy: yin and yang. Yin is your internal energy, whereas yang is the energy that allows you to be active in the world. You need a strong yin energy to be active (yang). If yin is depleted as from overwork or injury, then it is harder to be active (you will feel fatigued, depressed, or not want to get involved in activities). Acupuncture, in my opinion, is the best medicine to get you going again because it is so efficient in building yin. Massage, meditation, and yoga all complement the acupuncture treatment, so I usually recommend all.

6. Nourish the Adrenal Glands

I think the adrenals are the MOST important part of the body. They produce hormones such as estrogen, progesterone, DHEA, and testosterone. Everyone knows these are important, but few really know the impact the adrenals have via one more hormone: cortisol.

I discussed cortisol in Chapter 8. This is the hormone you need to make your best friend. Take good care of your adrenal cortisol like your life depended on it, because it does.

When the adrenal cortisol is "off" ANY kind of disease can manifest or get worse. I see it impact the gut, blood sugar, mood, inflammatory pathways, energy levels, and sleep in tremendous ways. If you are becoming imbalanced in any of these areas, you need to remember to treat the adrenals. Herbs work the best.

7. Avoid Processed Sugar

This food "group" is not good no matter how you try to justify it. Sugar seems to be in "everything" unless you are eating a whole food, unprocessed diet. Sugar promotes inflammation (Chapter 15) and is really hard on the body energetically (personal and clinical experience).

❧ 36 ❧

Prevention as "Cure"

1. Test Lipoprotein Levels

Conventional labs such as Lab Corps are now offering lipoprotein testing (Chapter 1) so you may specifically identify the types of cholesterol you have in your body. However, SpectraCell specialty lab had this test long before Lab Corps, so I tend to use this test instead as it is more specific and provides a patient data sheet showing treatments that work depending on the type of cholesterol you actually have.

I like to offer this test to my patients so we may then determine whether or not they are at risk of having low density LDLs in their system. If they do, then they need more aggressive antioxidant protection than a patient who does not. If their antioxidant level stays too low, they are at a higher risk of the developing atherosclerosis (Chapter 5). The low-density type of cholesterol particles are linked most directly to cardiovascular disease.

2. Keep Inflammation Low

This is very important because chronic diseases develop out of inflammation (clinical observation). I start with eliminating foods patients may be sensitive to. I also encourage them to reduce consumption of processed sugars (Johnson and Olefsky 2013).

Avoiding GMO (genetically modified food) is also key for keeping inflammation down. I do not have clinical trials to back this statement up, but I have seen in both myself and my patients that eating foods that are certified GMO free (you will see this on the label of the product) makes a big difference in symptom levels. According to Dr. Anderson, NMD (2011), GMO foods on the market increased "drastically since 1994" and include non-organic foods such as dairy, eggs, and wheat. As time goes by I am seeing increasing numbers of patients who can't eat any of these foods or they get sick. Some patients will show on their food tests that they are safe to eat the foods but if they do they feel bad. I am assuming it is because it is a GMO food.

Sugar in the diet promotes inflammation and bumps up HgA1c. I think that sugar may be a cause of autoimmune diseases, not to mention cancer. Don't eat any processed sugars for a few months and see how you feel. Then have some and see how you feel. I guarantee you will notice a big difference!

3. Keep a Positive Mind-set

If you are negative about your body and life, you will draw in negative experiences and poor health (Osteen 2005). The body will heal itself if the innate knowledge of healing is stimulated (Block 2011). This starts with the right mind-set. Work on minding your thoughts so they stay focused on what is good and right with your life.

4. Exercise

Exercise is the best way to feel great (other than eating well and maintaining a good attitude) and lower your risk of cancer (OncANP Conference 2013). Spending time in nature is key for healing according to research in the early 1980s by biologists Wilson and Ulrich (Simkovic 2013).

5. Support Your Adrenal Glands

I mentioned the adrenals in the previous chapter but I am going to do so again. Keep reading about these adrenals until the importance of what I am saying sinks in!

The adrenals in my opinion are the most important endocrine (hormone producing) gland in the body. They regulate sleep/wake cycle, mood, energy level, reproductive cycles, blood sugar, blood pressure, the immune system, and absorption of nutrients. Keep them healthy by keeping high levels of B Vitamins, Vitamin C, and magnesium in your diet and supplement regime. Then use herbs to nourish (such as Ashwagand-ha, Maca, or Rhodiola) and good amounts of sleep. The adrenals restore when you are sleeping. They also hold more Vitamin C in them than any other part of the body, which means they require high amounts of Vitamin C to make hormones.

I personally think most of our diseases (including cancer) are coming from a prob-lem with the adrenals. The adrenals regulate blood sugar. Elevated blood sugar we all know is connected to diabetes, but recent research is also showing it is connected to the creation of abnormal shifts within the immune system (Chapter 15). I have start-ed to test both fasting blood sugar and HgA1c (a chronic measure of high blood sugar levels) and in a vast majority of my patients I am finding NORMAL blood sugar but HIGH HgA1c.

Think about it. It means the blood sugar is elevating just enough for the body to store it but not enough that the body can't compensate for it yet (as shown by the normal fasting blood sugar). Technically, blood work like this means the patient is "pre-diabetic" but to me this means the patient is pre-cancer, pre-osteoarthritis, pre-fatty liver, pre-depression, pre-symptomatic menopause, pre-insomnia, pre-periph-eral neuropathy…need I go on?

I encourage you to read my mom's book, *Zip and Zap Take a Nap*. Zip and Zap show you how important taking care of your adrenals is. It is a children's book, but it is a great way to understand how important taking care of the adrenals are.

6. Genetic Testing of Detox Pathways

I like to use Genova Diagnostechs for my testing. They have tests for glutathione levels, oxidative damage, and polymorphisms (genetic abnormalities in detox pathways). If you know where you are weak genetically you can then use nutrition, herbs, and supplements to support your body so as to prevent chronic disease (Chapters 4 and 5).

7. Infrared Sauna

I like FIR infrared, available on Amazon.com. This wavelength of heat is just right for mobilizing toxins out of cells and excreted via the skin (Crinnion 2003-4). I recommend starting with 15 minutes a few times a week at a low heat setting. Some patients have adverse symptoms starting too hot too soon, for too long. Others have symptoms because their antioxidant levels are too low before they start the sauna, and when toxins begin to mobilize they get sick. If antioxidant levels are higher, the sauna will go better. After trying 5-10 minutes for a while, most patients are able to increase their time in the sauna.

8. Trust

Your body can heal itself—it has an amazing capacity to do so. The problem is that most physicians don't practice with that mind-set. In the words of Dr. Tallman, DC, NMD: "Your Body is a Healing Machine". He tells patients this while I tell them their body has an amazing ability to heal, and look how it already has done so. Give your body a chance to heal!

Part IV

Summary of Common Obstacles to Cure

This section is a summary of the most common causes of the most common diseases. Much of it is a repeat of what I have already discussed, but I wanted to provide a simple reference tool for you if you are seeking a quick reference to the identification of your medical conditions.

❧ 37 ❧
The Diseases and
Their Common Causes

**These are some of the most Common Diseases
and their Causes based on my experience:**

1. **Gallbladder Diseases**: Eggs and Irritable Bowel Syndrome

2. **Insomnia:** Elevated Cortisol, High Blood Sugar, an Unhappy Heart, Poor Liver Metabolism

3. **Depression:** Low a.m. Cortisol (Adrenal Dysfunction)

4. **Anxiety:** Adrenal Dysfunction

5. **Hot Flashes:** Sugar in Diet and Not Enough Liver Support

6. **Cervical Dysplasia:** Low Antioxidant Levels, Food Sensitivities, Negative Mind-set, Adrenal Fatigue, Exogenous Hormone Use, the HPV Vaccines

7. **Arthritis:** Gluten, Dairy, and Processed Sugars

8. **Swollen Joints:** Gluten and Dairy

9. **MS:** a Starving Mitochondria

10. **Painful Menstrual Cramps:** Gluten and Low Glutathione

11. **Irritable Bowel Syndrome:** Low 5-htp, Low Glutathione, Environmental Toxins, and Food Sensitivities

12. **Cancer:** Inflammation, Processed Sugar, Exogenous Hormone Intake, Environmental Toxins, Adrenal Dysfunction

13. **Fatty Liver:** Low Glutathione and IBS

14. **Fibromyalgia:** a Starving, Inflamed Mitochondria

15. **Peripheral Neuropathy:** Medication Side Effect and Gluten Intolerance

16. **UTIs:** Elevated Estrogen and Medication Side Effects

17. **Interstitial Cystitis:** Low Glutathione and Food Sensitivities

18. **Cracked Skin (especially at the Corners of Nails):** Low Antioxidant and Low Omega Oil Levels

19. **Memory Loss:** Too Many Bad Oils in the Diet

20. **Restless Legs:** Sugar, Liver Needs Support

21. **Agitated Feelings:** Sugar, Liver Needs Support

Naturopathic Medicine, when properly practiced, brings you into the "best version of yourself."
— AL, Flagstaff, AZ.

If you come to Naturopathic Medicine do NOT expect a quick fix. Naturopathy in and of itself is a journey. It's a journey of healing and of learning more about your self. It's also an investment in your self (financially).

Naturopathy is part of the Medicine of the Future because the Medicine of the Future will be focused on Identifying and Treating the Cause and Removing the Obstacles such that the body can heal. Someday, all physicians will be Naturopathic Doctors, or will be working closely with one. I may not live to see that day, but I am foreseeing this in our global future. There is a time and place for medications and surgery but they need to be in balance with Identification of the Cause.

Patients who work with me diligently to Identify their Causes or Obstacles, and treat those, start to feel really joyful and happy. I can't tell you how many times, during an acupuncture treatment for example, a patient said to me "I don't know what is happening to me but I feel so HAPPY!"

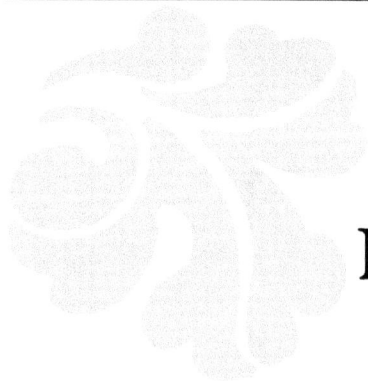

Part V

References

❧ 38 ❧
References

Abd El-Wahab, H. and Moram, G. "Toxic effects of some synthetic food colorants and/or flavor additives on male rats." **Toxicol Ind Health.** 2012. Feb 8.

American Psychiatric Association. **Diagnostic and Statistical Manual of Mental Disorders.** 2000. 4th ed.

Anderson, K., NMD. "Genetically Modified Food and Your Health." **Naturopathic Doctor News and Review.** January 2011. Vol. 7, Issue 1.

www.arizonaprolotherapy.com

Banerjee, P. **Chronic Disease.** Printed in India. 1931.

Block, D., ND, HMC. "Establishing the Mind-Body Connection in the Treatment of Autoimmune Illness." **Naturopathic Doctor News and Review.** March 2011. Vol. 7, Issue 3.

Boyle, W., ND and Saine, A., ND. **Lectures in Naturopathic Hydrotherapy.** Buckeye Naturopathic Press, East Palestine, Ohio. 1988.

Bonab, M. et al. "Autologous Mesenchymal Stem cell therapy in progressive multiple sclerosis: an open label study." **Curr Stem Cell Res Ther.** 2012. Oct 11.

Campbell, T and Campbell, T. **The China Study.** BenBella Books. 2006.

Carrasco-Valiente, J. et al. "State of acute phase markers and oxidative stress in patients with kidney stones in the urinary tract." **Actas Urol Esp.** 2012. May; 36(5): 296-301.

www.CDC.org

Champe, P. and Harvey, R. **Biochemistry.** Lippincott Williams and Wilkins, Philadelphia. 1994.

Crinnion, W., NMD. "Lectures in Environmental Medicine at Southwest College of Naturopathic Medicine." Tempe, AZ. 2003-5.

Davidson, S., DC, DO, ND. A **Popular Guide to Nature Cure.** D. B. Taraporevala Sons and Co. Private LTD, India. 1960.

DiPasquale, R., ND. "Using Low-Dose Herbs to Treat Pain." **Naturopathic Doctor News and Review.** 2009. Vol. 5, Issue 7.

Eder, C. "Mechanisms of IL-1B release." **Immunology.** 2009. Jul; 214(7):543-53.

www.edgarcayce.org/are/holistic_health/data/thcast1.html

www.en.wikipedia.org/wiki/Antioxidant

www.en.wikipedia.org/wiki/Cell_membrane

www.en.wikipedia.org/wiki/Glutathione

www.en.wikipedia.org/wiki/Obesity

www.en.wikipedia.org/wiki/File:USDA_Food_Pyramid.gif#file

Friedman, M., ND. "Autoimmune thyroid disease." **Naturopathic Doctor News and Review.** 2013. Volume 9, Issue 8.

Gao, Y. et al. "Effect of food azo dye tartrazine on learning and memory functions in mice and rats, and the possible mechanisms involved." **J Food Sci.** 2011. Aug; 76(6): T125-9.

Gowey, Brandie, NMD. **Your Cervix (Just) Has a Cold.** Morgan James, New York. 2014.

Greenspan, F. and Strewler, G. **Basic and Clinical Endocrinology.** Appleton and Lange, Stamford, CT. 1997.

Grotenhermen, F. and Russo, E. **Cannabis and Cannabinoids.** Routledge, London and New York. 2008.

Guyton, A. and Hall, J. **Textbook of Medical Physiology.** W.B. Saunders Co., Philadelphia. 2000.

Hahnemann, S. **The Chronic Diseases.** New Dehli, B. Jain Publishers, 1921.

Hask S. et al. "6-shagoal, a ginger product, modulator of neuroinflammation, a new approach to immunoprotection." **Neuropharmacology.** 2012. Aug; 6(2): 211-213.

www.healthchecksystems.com/antioxid.htm

Hoffer, A. **Healing Children's Attention and Behavior Disorders.** Toronto, Canada: CCNM Press Inc. 2005.

Horseen, S. et al. "The role of mitochondria in axonal degeneration and tissue repair in MS." **MS Journal.** 2012. 18(8): 1058-1067.

Huss, M., Völp, A., Stauss-Grabo, M. "Supplementation of polyunsaturated fatty acids, magnesium and zinc in children seeking medical advice for attention-deficit/

hyperactivity problems - an observational cohort study." **Lipids Health Dis.** 2010. Sep 24; 9:105.

Jansson, L., MD. "Infants of Mothers with Substance Abuse." **UpToDat.** Waltham, MA. 2014.

Jarrett, L. **Nourishing Destiny.** Spirit Path Press, Stockbridge, MA. 1998.

Johnson, A. and Olefsky, J. "The Origins and Drivers of Insulin Resistance." **Cell.** 2013. 152, February 14.

Kneipp, S. **My Water Cure.** Pilgrims Book PVT. LTD. Delhi. 1980.

Kim, J. et al." 6-gingerol suppresses interleukin-1 beta induced MUC5AC gene expression in human anway epithelial cells." **Am J Rhinol Allergy.** 2009. Jul-Aug; 23(4): 385-91.

Kroenke, C. et al. "High and low-fat dairy intake, recurrance, and mortality after breast cancer diagnosis." **J Nat'l Cancer Inst.** 2013.105(9): 616-623.

Krull, K. "Attention deficit hyperactivity disorder in children and adolescents: Overview of treatment and prognosis." In: **UpToDate.** Waltham, MA.2014.

Lord, R. and Fitzgerald, K. "Significance of Low Plasma Homocysteine." **Metametrix Clinical Laboratory.** Norcross, GA. 2006.

Lopez-Armada, M. et al. "Mitochondrial dysfunction and the inflammatory response." 2012 accepted manuscript.

Lyall, K. et al. "Maternal Dietary Fat Intake Associated with Autism Spectrum Disorders." **American Journal of Epidemiology.** 2013. 178(2): 209-220.

Meimaridou E. et al. "Renal oxidative vulnerability due to changes in mitochondrial-glutathione and energy homeostasis in a rat model of calcium oxalate urolithiasis." **Am J Physiol Renal Physiol.** 2006. Oct; 291(4): F731-40.

www.mdconsult.com/das/pdxmd/body/404981776-3/0?type=med&eid=9-u1.0-_1_mt_1014549).

www.mdconsult.com/das/search/results/403746318-13?searchId=1411701951&kw=UTI&area=FirstConsult&set=1&bbSearchType=single

www.mdconsult.com/das/pdxmd/body/403903122-12/1412416335?-type=med&eid=9-u1.0-_1_mt_1014469

www.mdconsult.com/das/pdxmd/body/403903122-13/1412417039?-type=med&eid=9-u1.0-_1_mt_5080901

www.mdconsult.com/das/pdxmd/body/402582560-4/1407380125?-type=med&eid=9-u1.0-_1_mt_1014218

www.mdconsult.com/das/search/results/403746318-9?searchId=1411691985&k-w=HTN&area=FirstConsult&set=1&bbSearchType=single

www.mdconsult.com/das/pdxmd/body/403746318-10/1411694919?-type=med&eid=9-u1.0-_1_mt_1014787

www.mdconsult.com/das/pdxmd/body/403746318-8/1411689153?-type=med&eid=9-u1.0-_1_mt_1014767

www.mdconsult.com/das/pdxmd/body/406922261-3/1424647993?-type=med&eid=9-u1.0-_1_mt_1014832

www.mdconsult.com/das/pdxmd/body/403746318-14/1411704308?-type=med&eid=9-u1.0-_1_mt_1014318

www.mdconsult.com/das/pdxmd/body/403903122-5/1412397058?-type=med&eid=9-u1.0-_1_mt_1014649

www.mdconsult.com/das/pdxmd/body/405943427-3/0?type=med&eid=9-u1.0-_1_mt_1014924

www.mdconsult.com/das/pdxmd/body/403903122-7/1412401531?-type=med&eid=9-u1.0-_1_mt_1014924

www.mdconsult.com/das/pdxmd/body/403903122-12/1412416335?-type=med&eid=9-u1.0-_1_mt_1014469

www.mdconsult.com/das/pdxmd/body/405943427-3/0?type=med&eid=9-u1.0-_1_mt_1014924

www.mdconsult.com/das/pdxmd/body/403903122-7/1412401531?-type=med&eid=9-u1.0-_1_mt_1014924

www.mdconsult.com/das/pdxmd/body/402582560-4/1407380125?-type=med&eid=9-u1.0-_1_mt_1014218

www.mdconsult.com/das/pdxmd/body/403903122-4/1412396832?-type=med&eid=9-u1.0-_1_mt_1014332

www.mdconsult.com/das/pdxmd/body/421094632-3/0?type=med&eid=9-u1.0-_1_mt_1016556

www.mdconsult.com/das/search/results/403746318-9?searchId=1411691985&k-w=HTN&area=FirstConsult&set=1&bbSearchType=single)

www.mdconsult.com/das/pdxmd/body/421209396-4/1467106703?-type=med&eid=9-u1.0-_1_mt_1014732

www.mdconsult.com/das/pdxmd/body/446973669-3/0?type=med&eid=9-u1.0-_1_mt_1014777

www.mdconsult.com/das/pdxmd/body/405410255-5/1418023963?-type=med&eid=9-u1.0-_1_mt_1014421).

www.mdconsult.com/das/pdxmd/body/403746318-10/1411694919?-type=med&eid=9-u1.0-_1_mt_1014787

www.mdconsult.com/das/pdxmd/body/403746318-8/1411689153?-type=med&eid=9-u1.0-_1_mt_1014767

www.mdconsult.com/das/search/results/403903122-9?searchId=1412406962&k-w=peripheral%20neuropathy&area=FirstConsult&set=1&bbSearchType=single

wwwmdconsult.com/das/pdxmd/body/406922261-3/1424647993?-type=med&eid=9-u1.0-_1_mt_1014832

www.mdconsult.com/das/pdxmd/body/403903122-6/1412398866?-type=med&eid=9-u1.0-_1_mt_1014742

www.mdconsult.com/das/pdxmd/body/403903122-3/1412396254?-type=med&eid=9-u1.0-_1_mt_1014339

www.mdconsult.com/das/pdxmd/body/403746318-3/0?type=med&eid=9-u1.0-_1_mt_1014435

Milte, C. et al. "Eicosapentaenoic and docosahexaenoic acids, cognition, and behavior in children with attention-deficit/hyperactivity disorder: a randomized controlled trial." **Nutrition.** 2012. Jun; 28(6): 670-7.

Murray, M. and Reutler, J. **Understanding Fats and Oils.** Apple Publishing, Vancouver. 1996.

Osteen, J. **Your Best Life Now.** Warner Faith, New York. 2005.

Oncology ANP conference on Breast Cancer, Keystone, CO. July 2013.

Pamphlett, R. "Exposure to environmental toxins and the risk of sporadic motor neuron disease: an expanded Australian case-control study." **Eur J Neurol.** 2012. Oct: 19(10): 1343-8.

Pellow J, et al. "Complementary and alternative medical therapies for children with attention-deficit/hyperactivity disorder (ADHD)." **Altern Med Rev.** 2011. Dec;16(4):323-37.

Ruiz, S. et al. "Targeting the transcription factor Nrf2 to ameliorate oxidative stress and inflammation in chronic kidney disease." **Kidney Int.** 2013. Jan 16.

Simkovic, V., ND. "Nature." **Naturopathic Doctor News and Review.** 2013. Vol. 9, Issue 3.

www.socialthinking.com

Soto, B. et al. "Impairment of intestinal glutathione synthesis in patients with inflammatory bowel disease." **Gut.** 1998. 42:485-492.

Steriti, R., ND, PhD. "The Calcium Controversy." **Naturopathic Doctor News and Review.** 2010. Vol. 6, Issue 10.

Substance Abuse and Mental Health Services Administration, **Results from the 2010 National Survey on Drug Use and Health: Summary of National Findings,** NSDUH Series H-41, HHS Publication No. (SMA) 11-4658. Rockville, MD: Substance Abuse and Mental Health Services Administration. 2011.

Swanson, M. "Gluten-free lyme whisperer." **Naturopathic Doctor News and Review.** 2013. Vol. 9, Issue 1.

Tallman, D., DC, NMD. "Severe Disc Extrusion and Resolution by Prolotherapy." **Naturopathic Doctor News and Review.** 2012. Vol. 8, Issue 11.

Tambouri, P., NMD. "Lectures in Urology Southwest College of Naturopathic Medicine." Tempe, AZ. 2005.

Thurton, L., ND. "Peripheral Neuropathy and Gluten: A Case Study." **Naturopathic Doctor News and Review.** 2013. Vol 9, Issue 7.

Tzekova, N. et al. "Molecules involved in the crosslink between immune and peripheral nerve Schwann cells." **J Clin Immunol.** 2014. Apr 17.

Waters, R., PhD. "Lectures in Genetics/Biochemistry Southwest College of Naturopathic Medicine." Tempe, AZ. 2003-4.

Wilens, T. et al. "Misuse and diversion of stimulants prescribed for ADHD: a systematic review of the literature." **J Am Acad Child Adolesc Psychiatry.** 2008. Jan;47(1):21-31.

Wodushek T. and Neumann, C. "Inhibitory capacity in adults with symptoms of Attention Deficit/Hyperactivity Disorder (ADHD)". **Arch Clin Neuropsychol.** 2003. Apr;18(3):317-30.

www.ingramcontent.com/pod-product-compliance
Lightning Source LLC
Chambersburg PA
CBHW060042030426
42334CB00019B/2444